The Homeostatic Reserve and Threshold Model

A Neurobiological Framework for Understanding Addictive Illness and Effective Treatment

Jeremy Mirabile, MD, ABPM-ADM, FASAM

Copyright and Publication Information

The Homeostatic Reserve Model, including its integrated definitions, propositions, visual architecture, and original educational figures, is the author's conceptual work. The component scientific concepts cited throughout the book have established independent histories and are not claimed as original by the author.

First edition, 2026.

Published by Awakening, Inc.

Paperback ISBN: 979-8-9972003-0-5. Hardcover ISBN: 979-8-9972003-1-2.

Interior design, typesetting, and production: Awakening, Inc.

Medical Disclaimer and Disclosures

This book is intended for professional education and general informational use. It does not establish a clinician–patient relationship, provide individual medical advice, replace a comprehensive diagnostic evaluation, or substitute for treatment by a qualified professional. Substance intoxication and withdrawal can be medically dangerous. A person with urgent symptoms, risk of overdose, severe withdrawal, suicidal thinking, psychosis, medical instability, or immediate danger should seek emergency evaluation.

Clinical standards, medications, regulations, occupational requirements, and levels of care change over time and vary by jurisdiction, diagnosis, patient characteristics, and setting. Readers should consult current authoritative guidance and exercise independent clinical judgment. References to ASAM, DSM, FAA, DOT, licensing, professional-health-program, confidentiality, and other standards are educational summaries and not legal, regulatory, or fitness-for-duty determinations.

The tank, threshold, zones, phases, curves, and trajectories in this book are conceptual educational representations. Homeostatic Reserve is not a biomarker, laboratory value, validated scale, DSM diagnosis, ASAM dimension, placement algorithm, or numerical predictor of recurrence.

The author is the developer of the Homeostatic Reserve Model and has professional interests in addiction treatment, education, speaking, and publication. This relationship is disclosed so readers can distinguish the author's original framework from the external scientific evidence cited throughout. No commercial product is endorsed by this book.

Clinical examples and patient statements are educational composites or generalized descriptions. They are not intended to identify any specific patient. Illness may help explain behavior, but it does not eliminate responsibility, safety requirements, accountability, or the need for repair where possible.

Introductory Note: The Question Behind This Book

Addiction is a chronic medical illness involving complex interactions among genetic susceptibility and resilience, environmental influences, trauma, stress, neuroplasticity, and dysregulation of the brain's motivational, reward, stress, learning, and executive-control systems. Yet clinicians, families, and patients continue to confront a fundamental question: Why does a person continue to use substances despite devastating consequences and a sincere desire to stop?

The question is often framed as a failure of knowledge, motivation, morality, or willpower. Those explanations are incomplete. Severe addictive illness can alter what captures attention, what feels urgent, what provides immediate relief, how strongly ordinary rewards motivate behavior, and how reliably the person can pause, integrate consequences, use support, and act according to long-term values.

This book develops an evidence-informed clinical framework for understanding that conflict. It integrates modern addiction neuroscience, multidimensional assessment, medication and psychosocial treatment, recovery capital, and more than two decades of clinical experience. The Homeostatic Reserve Model is introduced as a conceptual language for describing changing functional capacity—not as a biomarker or replacement for established diagnostic and placement standards.

The central clinical hope is practical: structured, evidence-based treatment can reduce destabilizing pressures, scaffold regulation, strengthen relationships, build trust with patients and families, and help restore enough capacity for healthy, value-consistent decisions to become possible again.

Preface

This book was written for clinicians, patients, families, educators, and professionals who need a scientifically grounded but clinically usable way to understand addictive illness. It begins with healthy motivation and regulation, follows the development and progression of illness, moves through comprehensive evaluation and treatment planning, and then examines recovery as a multidomain process extending beyond abstinence.

The Homeostatic Reserve Model arose from a recurring clinical observation: the same person may know what matters, value what matters, and act thoughtfully in one state, yet become much less able to live according to those values when withdrawal, stress, sleep loss, psychiatric symptoms, pain, cue exposure, isolation, or cumulative depletion intensify. The model proposes that changing integrated functional capacity helps explain why the fight can become profoundly unequal during severe illness and why treatment can make that fight more fair.

The model is intentionally broader than dopamine. Dopamine contributes to motivation, salience, learning, prediction, and effort, but the reserve represented by the tank also reflects biological stability, sleep, physical and psychiatric health, executive function, emotional regulation, coping, relationships, environment, natural reward, meaning, purpose, and hope. These domains do not function as independent ingredients. Their interaction creates the regulatory margin that is available to the person at a given time.

Throughout the book, established evidence is distinguished from clinical synthesis and from the author's original propositions. The figures are teaching tools, not validated instruments. The threshold is a conceptual boundary within the model, not a measured biological cutoff. The Healing Trajectory is a heuristic, not a universal timetable. These limits are essential to using the framework responsibly.

The language of the book is deliberately compassionate without abandoning accountability. A person can be profoundly impaired by illness and still require boundaries, safety, honesty, responsibility, and repair. Treatment does not create the patient's values. It helps restore the capacity to live by them.

Acknowledgments

This work is indebted first to the patients and families whose courage, suffering, persistence, and recovery have shaped the clinical questions explored in these pages. Their experiences repeatedly demonstrated that knowledge and values may remain present even when illness has made healthy action difficult to access.

I am grateful to the counselors, physicians, nurses, therapists, psychologists, case managers, peer-support professionals, monitoring professionals, and recovery communities whose work has shown how structure, medication, relationship, accountability, and time can help restore functioning. Special appreciation goes to the treatment team and staff at Recovery Keys—especially Jason Hunt, MD; Caitlin Labrador, LCSW; Ken DeBaun, CAC; Lisa Huser, CARN; Rebecca Caesar, RN; Chad Twyman; and Shanay Zackery—who help make quality treatment a reality every day.

I offer a specific acknowledgment to Joseph Jamison, CAC, an addiction counselor with whom I worked over many years. He brought Maslow's hierarchy into discussions of patients' healing journeys in treatment and helped keep questions of growth, meaning, and human potential present in the clinical conversation. I also want to acknowledge my colleague and friend, Jerry Gropper, DDS, LP, CAP, who introduced what I believe is the most effective way to treat this illness and helped me describe the process of treatment and recovery through his original work, *A Guide to Growing Up—Addiction Recovery*.

I also acknowledge the scientists and clinical organizations whose research and standards form the evidence base cited throughout the book. The Homeostatic Reserve Model is an original synthesis, but its component mechanisms depend on decades of work in neuroscience, medicine, psychology, recovery science, and public health.

Finally, I am grateful to the colleagues, friends, and family members who supported the long process of turning a clinical teaching framework into a manuscript.

Contents

List of Figures

All figures are original conceptual educational representations. Caption citations support component mechanisms; they do not validate the exact visual architecture of the Homeostatic Reserve Model.

PART I
FOUNDATIONS OF ADDICTIVE ILLNESS

Natural reward, vulnerability, disease development, and comprehensive evaluation

Part I moves from healthy regulation to vulnerability and then to the clinical task of determining severity, risk, and treatment need.

Chapter 1 — The Healthy Brain and Natural Reward

Homeostasis, Motivation, Choice, and the Capacity to Live According to Values

Before addictive illness can be understood, it is helpful to understand what healthy motivational and regulatory systems support. In healthy functioning, the brain does more than produce pleasure. Interacting systems help the person recognize needs, identify what matters, move toward beneficial experiences, avoid danger, learn from consequences, regulate internal states, maintain relationships, and adapt behavior over time.

Food, water, safety, attachment, achievement, intimacy, play, creativity, service, and meaning are often called natural rewards, but their function extends beyond enjoyment. They organize attention, learning, motivation, effort, social connection, and survival.

> *A healthy reward system does not simply help the person feel good. It helps the person recognize what is worth approaching, protecting, repeating, and becoming.*

Selected supporting evidence: [1–2,6–9].

Homeostasis

Homeostasis is the capacity of a living system to maintain sufficient internal stability while continuously adapting to changing demands. It does not mean that the body or mind remains motionless. Temperature, hunger, alertness, emotion, and stress activation all change. The healthy system repeatedly moves away from equilibrium and returns toward it.

A person with adequate regulation can experience hunger without becoming completely disorganized, disappointment without losing all hope, anxiety without requiring immediate escape, fatigue without abandoning every responsibility, and pleasure without needing it to continue indefinitely.

> *Homeostasis is not the absence of change. It is the capacity to move through change without losing the ability to regulate.*

Selected supporting evidence: [1–2].

Homeostatic Reserve

Within the Homeostatic Reserve Model, Homeostatic Reserve names the functional margin available when a person must regulate under stress, illness, emotional demand, or environmental challenge. Chapter 4 develops the formal definition and architecture.

Within the model, reserve reflects the combined functional influence of biological and psychiatric stability, sleep and circadian regulation, physical health and nutrition, cognitive and executive functioning, emotional regulation, natural reward responsiveness, learned coping, supportive relationships, environmental resources, meaning, purpose, and hope. No single component is the reserve. The construct represents the integrated functional result of these systems working together; it has not been validated as a single measurable quantity.

> *Reserve is the usable margin between current demands and the capacity available to meet them.*

The tank is a visual metaphor. Its apparent level should not be interpreted as a literal supply of dopamine, another neurotransmitter, willpower, morality, or a measurable biological fluid. Dopaminergic function contributes to motivation, salience, learning, effort, and reward responsiveness. Homeostatic Reserve is broader.

> *The tank represents capacity, not dopamine.*

Dopamine helps influence what feels important and worth pursuing. Within the model, Homeostatic Reserve describes the person's integrated capacity to regulate, adapt, recover, use support, experience natural reward, and act effectively. It cannot be inferred from a single neurotransmitter measure, PET finding, or receptor-availability estimate.

Supporting evidence for component mechanisms: [2–5]. The Homeostatic Reserve formulation is the author's conceptual synthesis and is not validated by these sources as a composite measure.

The Healthy Motivational System

Motivation begins with the detection of something important. A biological need, environmental cue, anticipated reward, danger, social signal, or remembered experience may attract attention and organize behavior.

Dopamine participates in salience, reward prediction, learning, motivation, effort, and the vigor with which an organism pursues an expected outcome. It should not be described simply as the brain's pleasure chemical.

> *Dopamine helps signal that something matters and may be worth pursuing. It does not, by itself, define happiness.*

A person may strongly want something without enjoying it proportionately. They may also enjoy an experience without developing an overwhelming drive to repeat it. Healthy motivation depends on coordination among multiple systems rather than one transmitter, receptor, or brain region.

Selected supporting evidence: [6–9].

Survival and Motivational Circuitry

The phrase reward center is useful for patient education but neurobiologically incomplete. Reward, salience, motivation, memory, stress, learning, habit, and executive control arise from interacting networks that include the ventral tegmental area, nucleus accumbens, dorsal striatum, prefrontal cortex, amygdala, hippocampus, insula, extended amygdala, and related systems.

In patient-facing language, these distributed networks may be described as survival and motivational circuitry or, more simply, the survival center. This is educational shorthand only—not a claim that one anatomical structure, transmitter, or receptor controls addiction.

> *The brain's motivational circuitry asks a basic question: What matters enough that I should direct attention, energy, learning, and behavior toward it?*

Figure 1.1 — The Healthy Reward and Regulation System

An integrated network of interacting systems that guide adaptive, value-congruent behavior.

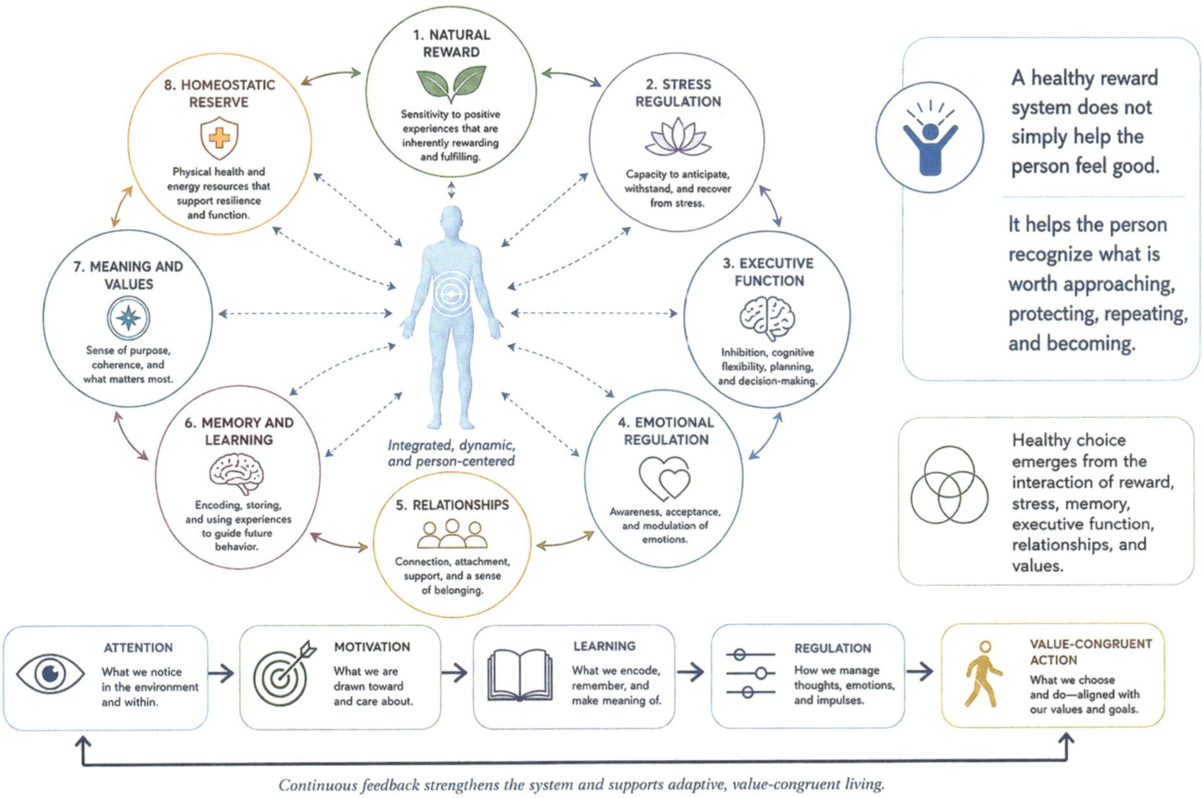

Figure 1.1. The Healthy Reward and Regulation System. Natural reward, stress regulation, executive function, emotional regulation, relationships, memory, meaning, values, and Homeostatic Reserve are shown as interacting influences on attention, motivation, learning, regulation, and value-congruent action. This figure is a conceptual educational representation, not a validated measurement instrument. Homeostatic Reserve represents integrated regulatory capacity, not a literal dopamine or neurotransmitter supply. Supporting evidence for component mechanisms: [1–2,6–7,11].

Selected supporting evidence: [9–11].

Natural Reward and Hedonic Tone

Natural rewards include food, water, rest, safety, affection, intimacy, play, exercise, mastery, creativity, recognition, service, spirituality, and meaningful contribution. A healthy life is not built from one reward. It is built from many moderate, varied, recurring sources of regulation and meaning.

Hedonic tone is a broad clinical construct describing the general capacity to experience pleasure, interest, positive emotional engagement, and reward from ordinary life. It is not constant happiness, a direct measure of dopamine, or a validated proxy for Homeostatic Reserve. A person with healthy hedonic tone can experience grief, boredom, disappointment, and distress while positive experiences remain sufficiently available to support participation in life.

Dopaminergic function contributes particularly to anticipation, motivational salience, willingness to exert effort, reinforcement learning, and translating expected reward into action. Hedonic tone also depends on opioid, endocannabinoid, serotonergic, glutamatergic, cortical, limbic, relational, and psychological systems. D2/D3 receptor availability in PET studies is influenced by multiple biological and methodological factors and should not be treated as a direct measure of dopamine level, pleasure, Homeostatic Reserve, or an individual patient's addiction severity.

Selected supporting evidence: [6,13–15].

Pavlovian Learning and Reinforcement

Learning allows the brain to anticipate important events and organize behavior before those events occur. In Pavlovian conditioning, a person, place, smell, sound, time of day, emotional state, or other previously neutral stimulus becomes associated with an important outcome. After repeated pairings, the cue itself may attract attention, create anticipation, activate physiological responses, or motivate approach.

> *The brain learns not only from the reward itself, but also from what reliably predicts it.*

Instrumental or operant learning occurs when behavior is shaped by what follows it. Positive reinforcement strengthens behavior because it produces a valued outcome. Negative reinforcement strengthens behavior because it reduces or removes an aversive state. Negative reinforcement is not punishment.

Pavlovian and instrumental learning often work together. A cue predicts an outcome, and the behavior that obtains or avoids that outcome becomes more likely. These normal learning processes later become central to addictive illness.

Selected supporting evidence: [16–18].

Figure 1.2 — Natural Reward, Reinforcement, and Learning

How cues, consequences, and learning guide adaptive behavior.

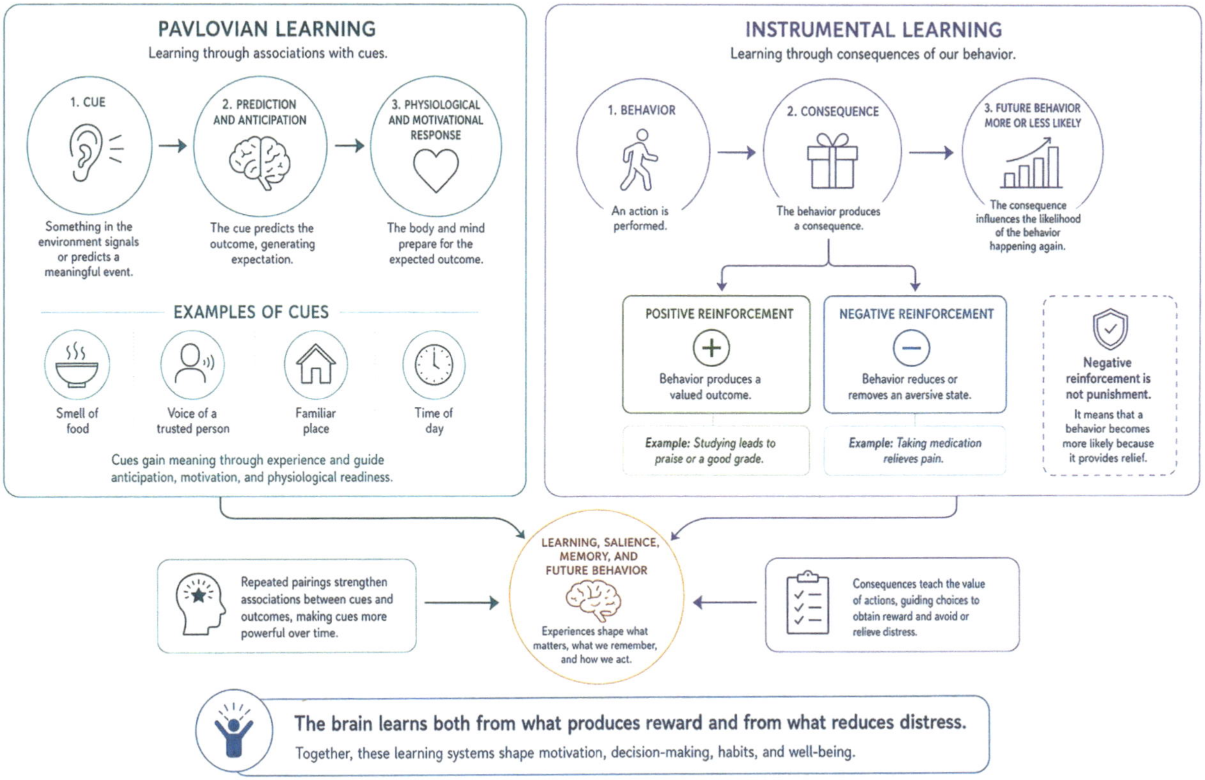

Figure 1.2. Natural Reward, Reinforcement, and Learning. Pavlovian learning links cues with predicted outcomes. Instrumental learning links behavior with consequences. Positive reinforcement produces a valued outcome; negative reinforcement provides relief from an aversive state. Supporting evidence for component mechanisms: [16–18].

Emotion, Stress, and Executive Function

Emotions provide information. Fear may signal threat, sadness may signal loss, anger may signal violation, guilt may signal behavior inconsistent with values, and joy may signal safety, connection, achievement, or fulfillment. Healthy regulation does not require suppressing these states. It involves recognizing them, tolerating them, interpreting them, and choosing how to respond.

> *Emotion is a signal. Regulation determines whether the signal becomes information or command.*

Stress systems are essential for survival. A healthy response is proportional, temporary, adaptive, and capable of resolving. Stress becomes destabilizing when demand draws on reserve faster than the person can restore it.

Executive functions support pausing, holding information in mind, inhibiting impulses, shifting strategies, planning, prioritizing, and organizing behavior around future goals.

> *Executive function creates time between urge and action.*

Within that time, the person may ask what is happening, what will follow, whether the action is consistent with values, whether help is needed, and whether another response is available.

Selected supporting evidence: [11,19–20].

Self-Awareness and Adaptive Course Correction

A healthy brain does more than pursue reward and avoid danger. It allows the person to observe behavior, compare intention with action, compare action with consequence, and compare current direction with the life they want.

Self-awareness is not perfect. Everyone has blind spots and may initially defend against painful information. Difficulty accepting illness occurs throughout medicine and psychiatry. A diagnosis may threaten identity, autonomy, professional role, family role, self-esteem, and the anticipated future.

Recognition requires the ability to observe evidence, tolerate its meaning, integrate it into an illness narrative, and allow it to change behavior.

Selected supporting evidence: [11,31].

Relationships, Mastery, Meaning, and Congruence

Human beings regulate partly through other people. A calm voice, trusted presence, honest conversation, comforting touch, shared routine, or sense of belonging can reduce stress and restore perspective.

Mastery develops through effort, feedback, practice, failure, correction, and eventual improvement. Competence teaches the brain that difficulty can lead to growth rather than requiring escape.

Meaning organizes behavior around something larger than immediate comfort. A person may tolerate substantial effort for a child, patient, relationship, vocation, spiritual commitment, community, or deeply held value.

> *Meaning gives the person a reason to tolerate discomfort without surrendering direction.*

Congruence occurs when thoughts, words, choices, and behavior increasingly align with values. Healthy regulation allows discomfort about incongruence to become a reason for correction rather than a reason for escape.

Selected supporting evidence: [58,89–90].

Maslow and the Homeostatic Threshold

Maslow's hierarchy offers a useful conceptual parallel for movement from physiological survival and safety toward belonging, esteem, self-actualization, and contribution. It should not be treated as a rigid staircase. Love, creativity, spirituality, and meaning can occur during adversity, but they are easier to sustain when regulation and safety are more secure.

> *The hierarchy does not describe human worth. It describes which forms of living become easier to sustain when basic regulation and safety are more secure.*

Within the Homeostatic Reserve Model, the Homeostatic Threshold is treated, for explanatory purposes, as a relatively stable conceptual boundary between broader value-congruent regulation and survival-oriented vulnerability. It is not a measured biological cutoff. Reserve is conceptualized as moving while the threshold provides a stable reference line.

The threshold is the line. Reserve is what moves.

Within the model, reflection, emotional regulation, natural reward, relationships, support, long-term values, and adaptive choice are conceptualized as more reliably available above the threshold. Below it, immediate relief and survival-oriented behavior may become increasingly dominant. This is a probabilistic shift, not an absolute switch.

Figure 1.3 — Homeostatic Reserve in Healthy Regulation

Reserve falls under stress and recovers through restorative processes.

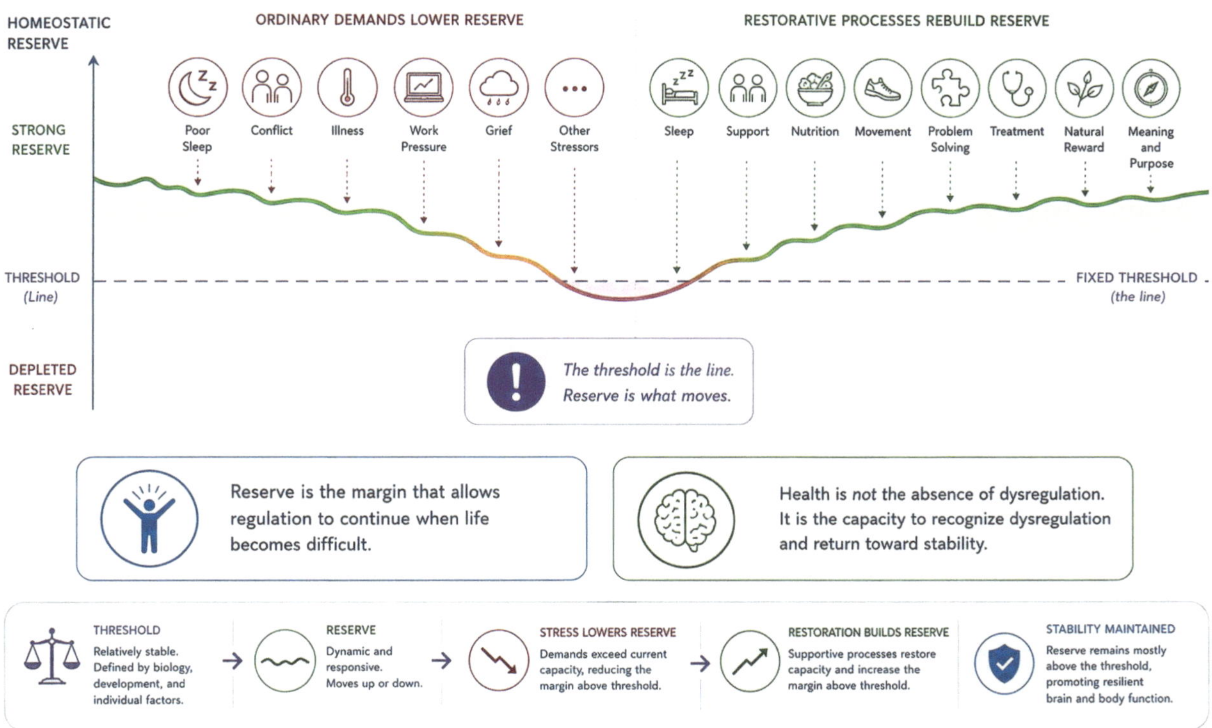

Healthy regulation is a cycle: notice, respond, restore, and return toward stability.

Figure 1.3. Homeostatic Reserve in Healthy Regulation. Ordinary demands may temporarily lower reserve, while sleep, support, nutrition, movement, problem solving, treatment, natural reward, and meaning may help restore it. Health is represented as the capacity to recognize dysregulation and return toward stability. The tank, threshold, and directional changes are conceptual educational representations, not validated measurements or biological cutoffs. Homeostatic Reserve represents integrated regulatory capacity, not a literal dopamine or neurotransmitter supply. Supporting evidence for component mechanisms: [1–3].

Supporting evidence for component mechanisms: [2,82–83]. These sources support component mechanisms; the model's integrated relationship remains an original conceptual proposition.

Chapter 1 Closing Perspective

Healthy functioning depends on coordinated systems that keep natural reward, emotion, relationships, and long-term values available under stress. Chapter 2 follows what can happen when vulnerability, intense relief, learning, and repeated exposure begin to reorganize those systems.

A healthy reward system helps the person recognize not only what feels good, but what is worth protecting.

Chapter Summary

Healthy regulation emerges from coordinated systems that support natural reward, homeostasis, learning, emotional regulation, executive function, relationships, and meaning. Within the Homeostatic Reserve Model, their interaction creates the functional margin that allows a person to adapt under stress without losing access to long-term values.

Key Clinical Takeaways

- Dopamine contributes to salience, prediction, motivation, learning, and effort; it is not synonymous with pleasure, happiness, or Homeostatic Reserve.
- The tank represents integrated functional capacity, not a neurotransmitter supply.
- Executive function creates time between urge and action, while relationships and meaning help organize behavior beyond immediate comfort.
- The Homeostatic Threshold is a conceptual boundary within the model; it is not a measured biological cutoff.

Chapter 2 — Vulnerability, Stress, and the Development of Addictive Illness

How Healthy Motivational Systems Become Organized Around Relief and Survival

Addictive illness does not begin in the same way for every person. Some individuals have substantial inherited, developmental, psychiatric, or medical susceptibility before first exposure. For others, prolonged stress, trauma, pain, intense reinforcement, repeated exposure, environmental availability, or substance potency may contribute more strongly. For many patients, several pathways interact, and no single pathway is necessary or sufficient in every case.

> *Addictive illness develops through the interaction of vulnerability, exposure, stress, learning, and adaptation over time.*

The illness does not develop because the patient lacks values, goodness, or concern for others. It develops when powerful reinforcement, conditioned learning, stress, neuroadaptation, and repeated substance exposure increasingly recruit brain systems responsible for motivation, regulation, and survival.

Selected supporting evidence: [10,21–23,25].

People Do Not Begin With the Same Reserve

Within the Homeostatic Reserve Model, inherited biology, prenatal and early development, temperament, attachment, trauma, nutrition, sleep, physical health, neurodevelopmental conditions, psychiatric illness, social stability, and early experiences of reward and stress may influence baseline regulatory capacity. Baseline reserve is a conceptual construct, not a validated score.

Two people may be exposed to the same substance and experience very different effects. One may find it pleasant but limited. Another may experience unusually powerful relief, calm, energy, confidence, focus, connection, or emotional normality.

> *The same substance may enter two different nervous systems and acquire two very different meanings.*

Selected supporting evidence: [2,21,25–26].

Genetic and Biological Susceptibility

Substance-use disorders have a substantial heritable component at the population level, but addictive illness should not be described as beginning from one universal genetic vulnerability. Every person has a biologically and genetically shaped nervous system, while the magnitude, mechanisms, and clinical importance of inherited susceptibility vary by disorder, population, environment, and individual.

The relative contribution of inherited vulnerability differs substantially. In some patients, genetic liability may be prominent. In others, developmental adversity, psychiatric or medical illness, repeated exposure, environmental conditions, or substance potency may contribute more strongly to the observed trajectory. Addiction is therefore best understood as the product of interacting susceptibilities and exposures rather than one universal genetic origin.

Everyone has a biologically shaped susceptibility. Not everyone begins with the same degree of inherited vulnerability.

Genetic influences may affect reward sensitivity, stress reactivity, impulsivity, temperament, metabolism, subjective response, executive function, psychiatric vulnerability, and reinforcement learning. Genes influence the terrain; development, exposure, stress, potency, access, and learning help determine the path taken across it.

Selected supporting evidence: [21–22].

Developmental Vulnerability, Trauma, and Chronic Stress

The brain develops within relationships and environments. Early experiences may influence emotional regulation, attachment, expectations of safety, trust, stress tolerance, self-soothing, and the ability to use support. These associations are probabilistic and do not determine an individual outcome.

A child exposed to instability, neglect, violence, inconsistent caregiving, chronic fear, or humiliation may develop adaptations that increase vigilance or prepare the nervous system for danger. Such adaptations may be protective in the original environment and may carry later costs, but trauma history does not produce one uniform neurobiological or clinical course.

A nervous system shaped for survival may remain highly effective at detecting threat while having greater difficulty experiencing safety.

Trauma may include both events and their lasting effects on regulation, memory, identity, and safety. Chronic stress may also be depleting: caregiving burden, poverty, occupational pressure, unstable housing, pain, conflict, discrimination, sleep disruption, and persistent medical illness. The effect of any exposure varies with timing, intensity, duration, context, protective factors, and the individual.

Selected supporting evidence: [23–25].

Psychiatric and Medical Vulnerability

Depression, anxiety, bipolar disorder, trauma-related disorders, ADHD, obsessive-compulsive symptoms, eating disorders, psychotic illness, personality-related dysregulation, and neurocognitive conditions may increase vulnerability or consume regulatory capacity before substance use begins. Relationships are bidirectional: psychiatric symptoms may increase substance-use risk, and substances may worsen, mimic, or complicate psychiatric illness.

The patient may initially use to regulate panic, insomnia, racing thoughts, depression, intrusive memories, shame, social anxiety, irritability, or emotional numbness.

The substance may initially appear to treat a symptom before it becomes part of a larger illness.

Medical illness and pain may consume regulatory capacity through disrupted sleep, mood, mobility, work, relationships, attention, and hope. A substance or medication that rapidly relieves pain or distress may acquire substantial motivational value, although trajectories vary and appropriate medical treatment should not be conflated with addictive illness.

A legitimate search for relief can become captured by a system that progressively narrows freedom.

Selected supporting evidence: [25–26,92].

Low Hedonic Tone and Borrowed Normality

Some patients describe ordinary life before substantial exposure as emotionally flat, effortful, disconnected, or insufficiently motivating. For some, a powerful early substance effect may feel less like intoxication and more like what this model calls borrowed normality. This is a clinical description within the Homeostatic Reserve Model, not a validated phenotype or proof of a specific premorbid neurochemical deficit.

> *For some patients, a powerful substance effect may feel less like intoxication and more like borrowed normality.*

The patient may experience calm for the first time, energy without overwhelming effort, confidence without fear, focus without constant struggle, connection without self-consciousness, or relief without waiting. They may think, "I finally feel like myself."

Within the model, the state is called borrowed because the experience is produced by an externally delivered, non-sustainable regulator rather than by stable health, relationships, coping, and varied natural reward. The term does not imply that every patient began with the same deficit or that the substance corrected a known biological abnormality.

Selected supporting evidence: [6,13,26–27].

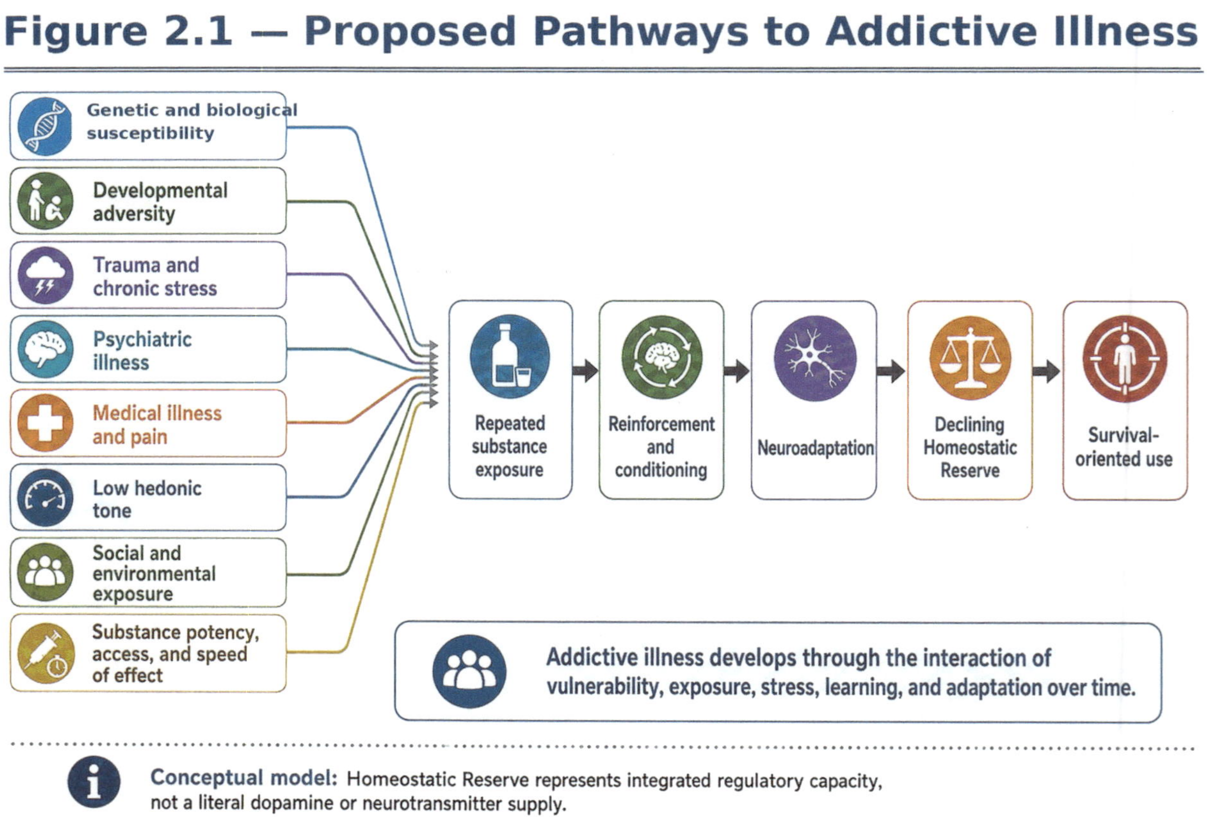

Figure 2.1. Proposed Pathways to Addictive Illness. This conceptual model integrates evidence on genetic and biological susceptibility, development, stress, psychiatric and medical burden, low hedonic tone, substance exposure, reinforcement, conditioning, and neuroadaptation within the Homeostatic Reserve framework. Individual susceptibility reflects interacting biology, development, environment, and exposure; no single pathway is necessary or sufficient in every patient. This figure is a conceptual educational representation, not a validated causal map, risk score, or measurement instrument. Homeostatic Reserve represents integrated regulatory capacity, not a literal dopamine or neurotransmitter supply. Supporting evidence for component mechanisms: [21,23,25–27].

Exposure, Potency, and Speed of Effect

Susceptibility alone does not produce substance-related illness. Exposure matters. Frequency, potency, route, speed of onset, duration, availability, affordability, and the reliability with which the substance changes the internal state influence reinforcement.

> *The faster and more reliably a substance changes the internal state, the more strongly the brain may learn to return to it.*

A person with substantial vulnerability may never develop illness without meaningful exposure. Intense or prolonged exposure to a highly reinforcing substance may produce illness in someone without a striking family history or obvious premorbid vulnerability.

Selected supporting evidence: [9,12,27].

From Relief Seeking to Survival Seeking

Early use may involve what the model calls borrowed normality, pleasure, curiosity, belonging, confidence, energy, reduced inhibition, or emotional ease. Positive reinforcement can strengthen behavior because it produces a valued effect.

For some patients, motivation may shift over time from seeking pleasure or relief toward avoiding withdrawal, anxiety, dysphoria, insomnia, pain, shame, loneliness, irritability, trauma-related distress, boredom, or emotional emptiness. The sequence, timing, and degree of this shift vary by substance and individual.

Negative reinforcement is not punishment. It means behavior becomes stronger because it reduces an aversive state.

> *What begins as a pursuit of reward may become a learned escape from suffering.*

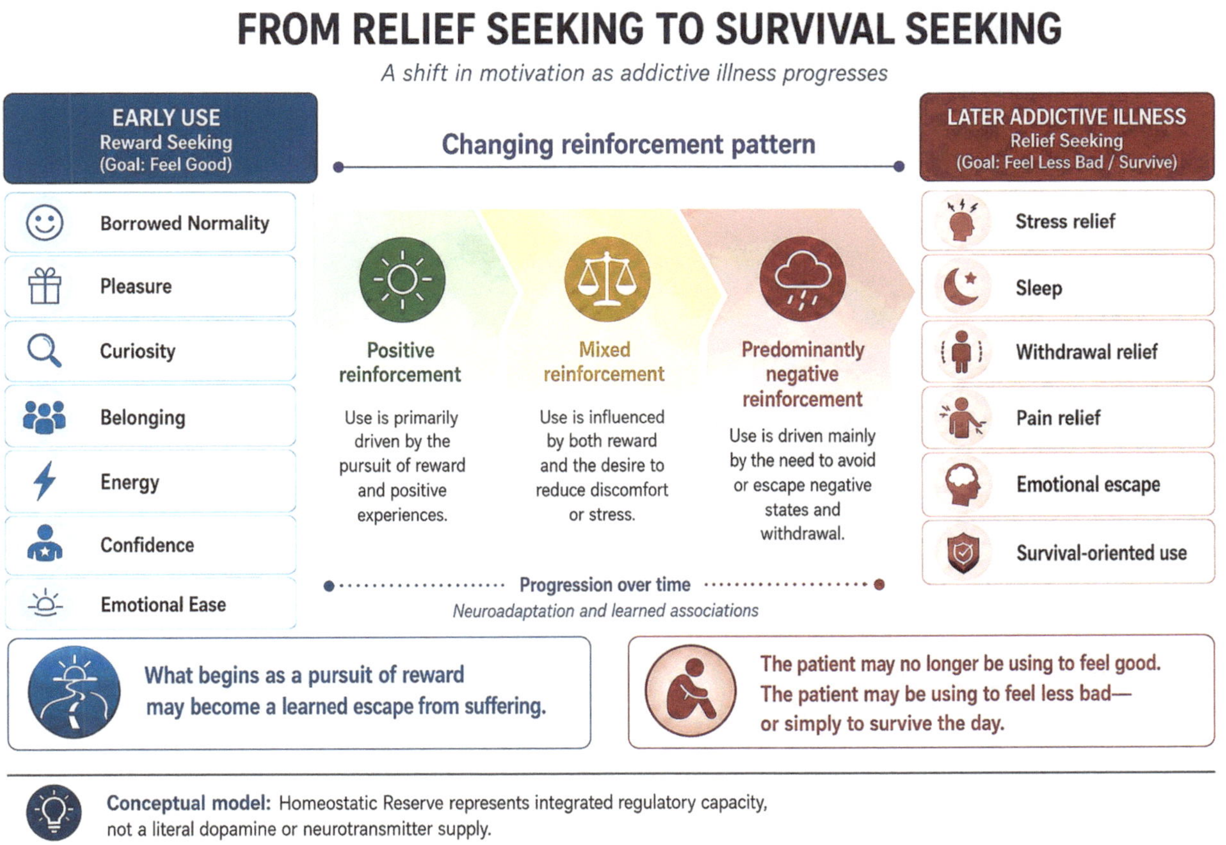

Figure 2.2. From Relief Seeking to Survival Seeking. Within the Homeostatic Reserve Model, motivation may shift from early reward or borrowed normality toward mixed and then predominantly negative reinforcement, including withdrawal relief, stress reduction, sleep, pain relief, and emotional escape. This is a conceptual educational progression, not a validated stage sequence or a universal course. Homeostatic Reserve represents integrated regulatory capacity, not a literal dopamine or neurotransmitter supply. Supporting evidence for component mechanisms: [28–29,51].

Selected supporting evidence: [10,28–30,51].

The Substance Becomes a Regulator

As use continues, the substance may become a primary regulator. It may be used to wake up, calm down, sleep, socialize, work, tolerate pain, suppress memory, reduce fear, celebrate, grieve, or feel anything at all.

> *The problem is not only that the patient uses the substance. The problem is that more and more of life becomes organized around needing it to regulate.*

Healthy coping is flexible. Addictive illness progressively concentrates regulation into one powerful method. The narrower the repertoire, the greater the vulnerability when the substance is unavailable.

Selected supporting evidence: [10,25,28].

Pavlovian Conditioning and Instrumental Learning

Repeated use teaches the brain not only about the substance but about everything that predicts it. Through Pavlovian conditioning, people, places, smells, sounds, routes, objects, emotional states, and times of day acquire motivational significance.

> *The brain learns not only the substance, but the entire world that predicts the substance.*

Instrumental learning strengthens behaviors that obtain the substance or reduce distress. Calling a particular person, visiting a location, carrying cash, concealing information, or withdrawing from family may become efficient, practiced sequences.

Selected supporting evidence: [16–17,84–85].

Neuroadaptation and Progressive Narrowing

The nervous system may adapt to repeated exposure. Depending on the substance, pattern of use, and patient, tolerance, withdrawal, altered reward responsiveness, stress-system dysregulation, cue sensitivity, habit formation, and less reliable executive control may develop. Some patients require more substance for the same effect while ordinary life becomes less rewarding; these changes are heterogeneous and may improve to differing degrees during recovery.

This is not a literal emptying of dopamine. Within the model, a decline in reserve means that the combined capacity for reward responsiveness, stress regulation, executive control, emotional tolerance, physical stability, relationships, and adaptive action has become less reliable. It is a conceptual functional description, not a directly measured neurochemical state.

Salience determines what stands out as important. Substance cues and relief may acquire disproportionate salience, while family, work, health, and meaning remain intellectually important but lose motivational force.

> *The patient may still know what matters while becoming less able to feel its importance strongly enough to guide behavior.*

Selected supporting evidence: [10–12,18].

Crossing the Threshold and the Unfair Fight

Continued intoxication, withdrawal, insomnia, poor nutrition, psychiatric symptoms, pain, secrecy, shame, conflict, financial strain, cue exposure, and repeated crisis may lower reserve. Within the Homeostatic Reserve

Model, as reserve approaches the conceptual threshold, urgency, rigidity, isolation, cue-driven behavior, defensiveness, and resistance to help may increase.

The lower the reserve, the more immediate relief can dominate the field of choice.

Within the model, healthy capacities remain present below the threshold but may become less available and less reliable. The patient may know what matters while feeling compelled toward immediate relief. This is a probabilistic shift, not an absolute loss of agency.

Within the Homeostatic Reserve Model, active addictive illness can create an unfair fight between immediate, conditioned, survival-oriented relief and healthy behaviors whose benefits are slower, less certain, and harder for the patient to feel.

Patients often say, "I do not want to use, but I feel like I need it." This is not a simple contradiction. It reflects conflict among values, executive knowledge, conditioned motivation, withdrawal, relief seeking, and depleted reserve.

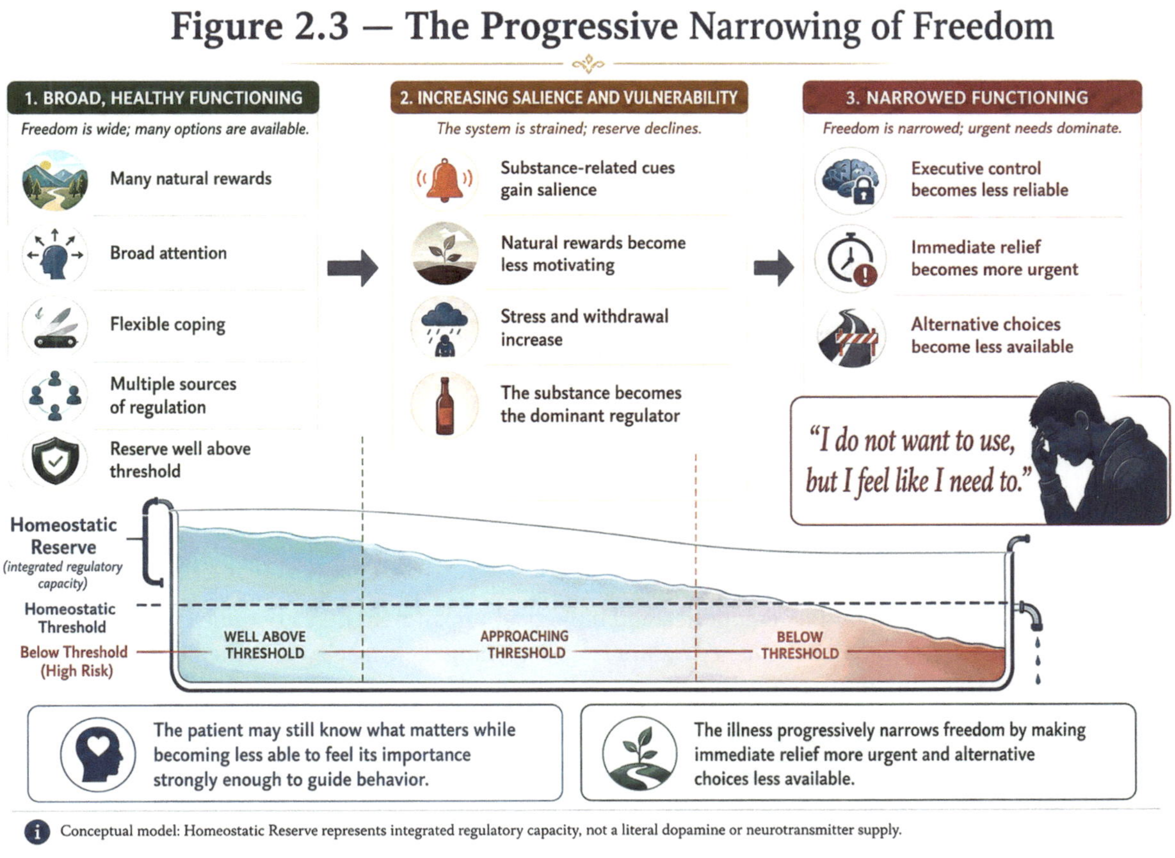

Figure 2.3. The Progressive Narrowing of Freedom. Within the model, substance-related salience, conditioned cues, stress, withdrawal, habit, and declining reserve may progressively narrow available freedom of action. Natural rewards may lose motivational force while immediate relief gains disproportionate influence. This figure is a conceptual educational representation, not a validated measurement of freedom, reserve, threshold position, or individual prognosis. Homeostatic Reserve represents integrated regulatory capacity, not a literal dopamine or neurotransmitter supply. Supporting evidence for component mechanisms: [10–12,18].

Supporting evidence for component mechanisms: [10–11,19,51]. These sources support component mechanisms; the model's integrated relationship remains an original conceptual proposition.

Why the Illness Can Be Difficult to Recognize

Addictive illness may impair judgment, insight, memory, salience, self-monitoring, emotional tolerance, and executive control—the capacities needed to recognize illness and organize life around care. Impaired insight should be distinguished from ordinary psychological defense, shame, ambivalence, incomplete memory, cultural or relational context, and intentional concealment.

> *The organ being asked to recognize the illness is itself affected by the illness.*

Denial may begin as a human defense against painful reality. Addiction can add the central contradiction that the substance has become both a cause of suffering and a rapidly available source of relief. No single explanation accounts for every patient's minimization, omission, or resistance.

The patient may recognize every consequence separately while remaining unable to recognize the illness connecting them. Repeated consequences may gradually weaken explanations that protect denial, but treatment should help make the pattern visible before catastrophe is required.

Selected supporting evidence: [11,31].

A Good Person With a Powerful Illness

Behaviors during active illness may be far from the patient's values. The patient may lie, isolate, break commitments, misuse medication, or behave in ways that produce pain. The illness can help explain impaired capacity without excusing harm. Recovery requires honesty, responsibility, safety, changed behavior, and repair where possible; the behavior still does not define the whole person.

> *The patient is a person with a powerful illness—and remains responsible for safety, accountability, and repair.*

Selected supporting evidence: [73–74].

Early Recovery and Scaffolding

After substance cessation, cognitive, emotional, and biological impairment may continue beyond acute withdrawal. Some patients regain abstinence before fully regaining the capacity to make healthy decisions reliably; the degree and duration of impairment vary and should be assessed rather than presumed.

A structured environment may provide sleep, meals, indicated medication, therapy, monitoring, reduced access, and predictable routines. Indicated medications may reduce specific pressures such as withdrawal, craving, autonomic distress, psychiatric symptoms, pain, or sleep disruption. Effects vary by diagnosis, medication, adherence, patient, and setting.

Supporting evidence for component mechanisms: [34,36–37,63]. These sources support component mechanisms; the model's integrated relationship remains an original conceptual proposition.

Integrating the Three Figures

Taken together, Figures 2.1 through 2.3 illustrate one proposed progression from vulnerability to illness. Figure 2.1 shows multiple converging pathways. Figure 2.2 shows a possible motivational shift from early reward or relief toward survival-oriented use. Figure 2.3 shows how conditioning, salience, stress, withdrawal, and declining reserve may progressively narrow freedom. The figures are related conceptual teaching tools, not validated stages or a universal natural history.

The substance may begin as pleasure—or as an attempt to change an uncomfortable internal state. For some patients it may provide what this model calls borrowed normality, then become relief, and eventually be experienced as necessary for survival. Other patients follow different pathways.

Selected supporting evidence: [10–12,18].

Chapter 2 Closing Perspective

> *What begins as an attempt to feel better may become an illness organized around avoiding feeling worse.*

Once relief has become a dominant regulator, the next clinical task is to determine the illness's present severity, functional impact, risks, and level-of-care needs.

Chapter Summary

Addictive illness develops through interacting vulnerability, exposure, reinforcement, conditioning, stress, and neuroadaptation. Early use may provide pleasure or borrowed normality, but repeated exposure can shift behavior toward negative reinforcement, survival-oriented relief, and progressive narrowing of freedom.

Key Clinical Takeaways

- Genetic, developmental, psychiatric, medical, and environmental influences alter risk without determining an individual outcome.
- Borrowed normality is a clinical description of an experience, not a validated biological subtype.
- The motivational shift from reward seeking toward relief seeking is common but not universal or strictly staged.
- Severe illness can create an unfair fight between immediate conditioned relief and healthy alternatives whose benefits are slower to feel.

Chapter 3 — Evaluating Addictive Illness

Diagnosis, Severity, Level of Care, Cognition, and Clinical Synthesis

A comprehensive evaluation of addictive illness must do more than determine whether diagnostic criteria are present. It should describe what the illness is doing now: intoxication and withdrawal risk, addiction-medication needs, biomedical conditions, psychiatric and cognitive conditions, substance-use-related risks, recovery-environment interactions, person-centered considerations, functional loss, and the intensity and type of services required.

> *Diagnosis names the illness. Evaluation determines what the illness is doing now and what treatment must do next.*

Selected supporting evidence: [32–33].

Diagnosis, Placement, and Clinical Synthesis

Three related but distinct tasks are required: establish diagnoses; assess multidimensional risks, needs, strengths, and resources; and integrate the findings into an individualized plan for level of care, medication, monitoring, and continuing treatment.

A diagnosis does not automatically determine level of care. Symptom count alone does not establish low risk when significant intoxication or withdrawal, biomedical or psychiatric instability, cognitive impairment, substance-use-related risk, an unsafe recovery environment, or safety-sensitive work is present.

Clinical synthesis asks not merely whether the patient meets criteria, but how much freedom, regulation, health, cognition, and safety the illness has taken.

Selected supporting evidence: [32–33,94].

A Multidimensional Assessment

The ASAM Criteria, Fourth Edition, organizes assessment across six dimensions and their subdimensions: Intoxication, Withdrawal, and Addiction Medications; Biomedical Conditions; Psychiatric and Cognitive Conditions; Substance Use-Related Risks; Recovery Environment Interactions; and Person-Centered Considerations. Dimensions 1 through 5 inform the initial clinically indicated level-of-care recommendation through the Dimensional Admission Criteria. Dimension 6 then supports shared decision-making about where the patient is willing and able to engage. Risk ratings should not be averaged into a universal severity score.

> *Patient preference matters and is central to shared decision-making, but it does not convert an unsafe or clinically inadequate option into the clinically indicated level of care.*

The level-of-care assessment should address the six Fourth Edition dimensions. A fuller treatment-planning assessment should also identify priorities, strengths, resources, barriers, motivational needs, co-occurring conditions, and the services needed at or alongside the recommended level of care. Reassessment should guide continued service and transitions as needs change.

Selected supporting evidence: [32,92].

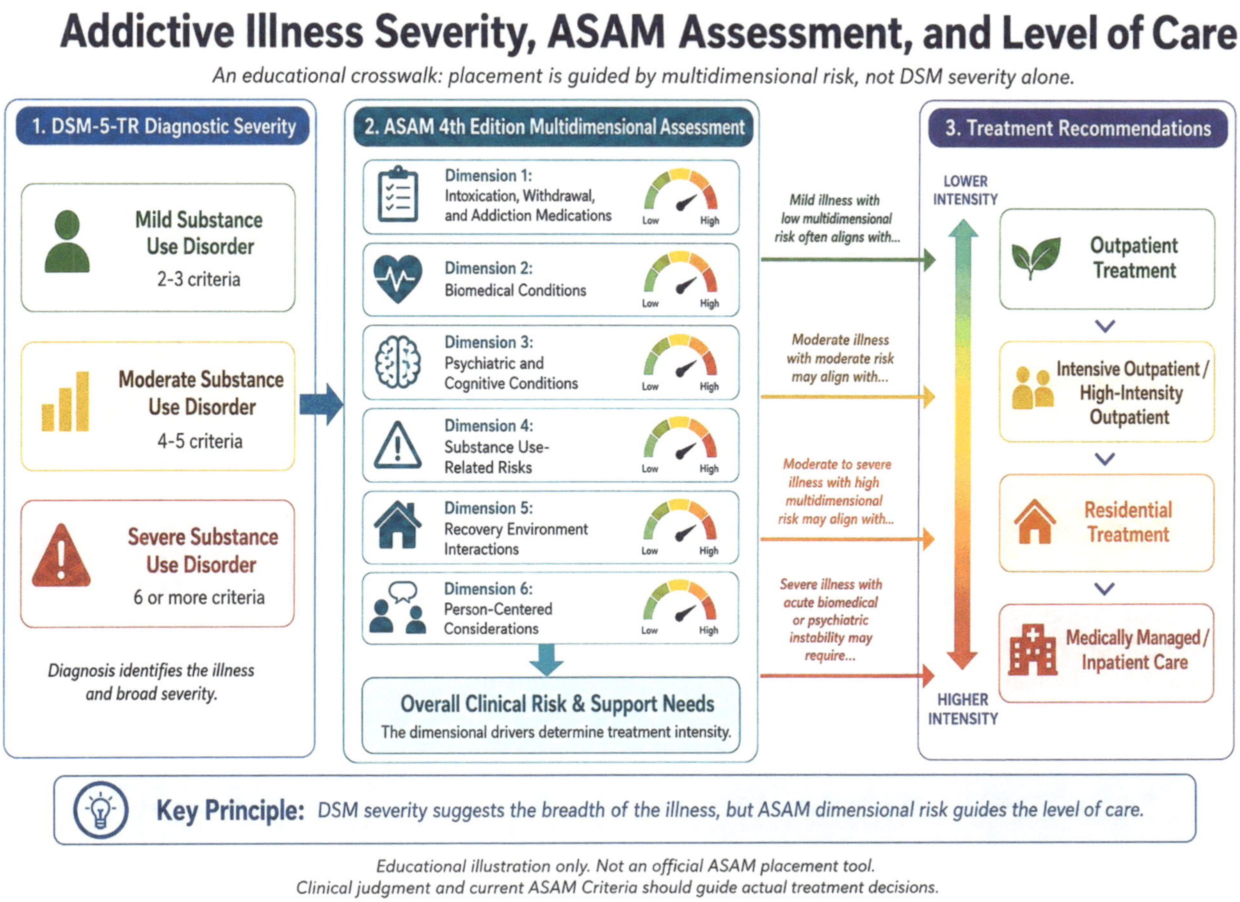

Figure 3.1. Assessment and Care-Level Integration. Diagnosis, the ASAM Criteria Level of Care Assessment, application of Dimensional Admission Criteria, shared decision-making, treatment planning, and reassessment are related but distinct tasks. This is a conceptual educational summary, not a substitute for The ASAM Criteria, its proprietary algorithms, or individualized clinical judgment. Supporting evidence for component mechanisms: [32–33].

Withdrawal and Biological Risk

The evaluator should determine whether the patient is intoxicated, entering withdrawal, expected to experience clinically significant withdrawal, in need of initiation or titration of addiction medication, or medically unstable. Risk may change rapidly and can require medical evaluation, monitoring, medication, and a level of care capable of managing anticipated complications.

For patients at clinically significant risk, medication-assisted withdrawal management during the detoxification phase may reduce suffering, prevent complications, and create enough stability for participation in comprehensive treatment. The appropriate setting and medication depend on substance, severity, comorbidity, prior withdrawal history, and current clinical findings.

> *Withdrawal management creates safety and stability. It does not, by itself, constitute treatment of the addictive illness.*

The clinician must also evaluate pain, sleep disorders, nutrition, pregnancy, neurologic disease, medication interactions, endocrine problems, infection, cardiopulmonary illness, and other conditions that may alter risk or capacity.

Selected supporting evidence: [34–36].

Psychiatric and Cognitive Evaluation

Mood instability, anxiety, psychosis, attentional problems, dissociation, sleep disturbance, personality-like behavior, and cognitive impairment may reflect a primary disorder, a substance-induced syndrome, intoxication, withdrawal, sleep loss, trauma activation, or several interacting causes.

Initial diagnoses may need to remain provisional. Serial observation during stabilization can clarify whether symptoms resolve, improve partially, or persist independently. Clinicians should neither presume that symptoms are substance-induced nor prematurely assume that every presentation represents an enduring primary disorder.

> *A diagnosis made during severe dysregulation may describe the presentation accurately without yet identifying its enduring cause.*

Brief cognitive screening can identify concern but may not adequately evaluate executive function, memory, attention, processing speed, visuospatial ability, or complex decision-making. When cognition affects treatment participation, informed decision-making, return to work, or public safety, comprehensive domain-specific neuropsychological testing and expert interpretation may be required.

Selected supporting evidence: [33,47–50,92].

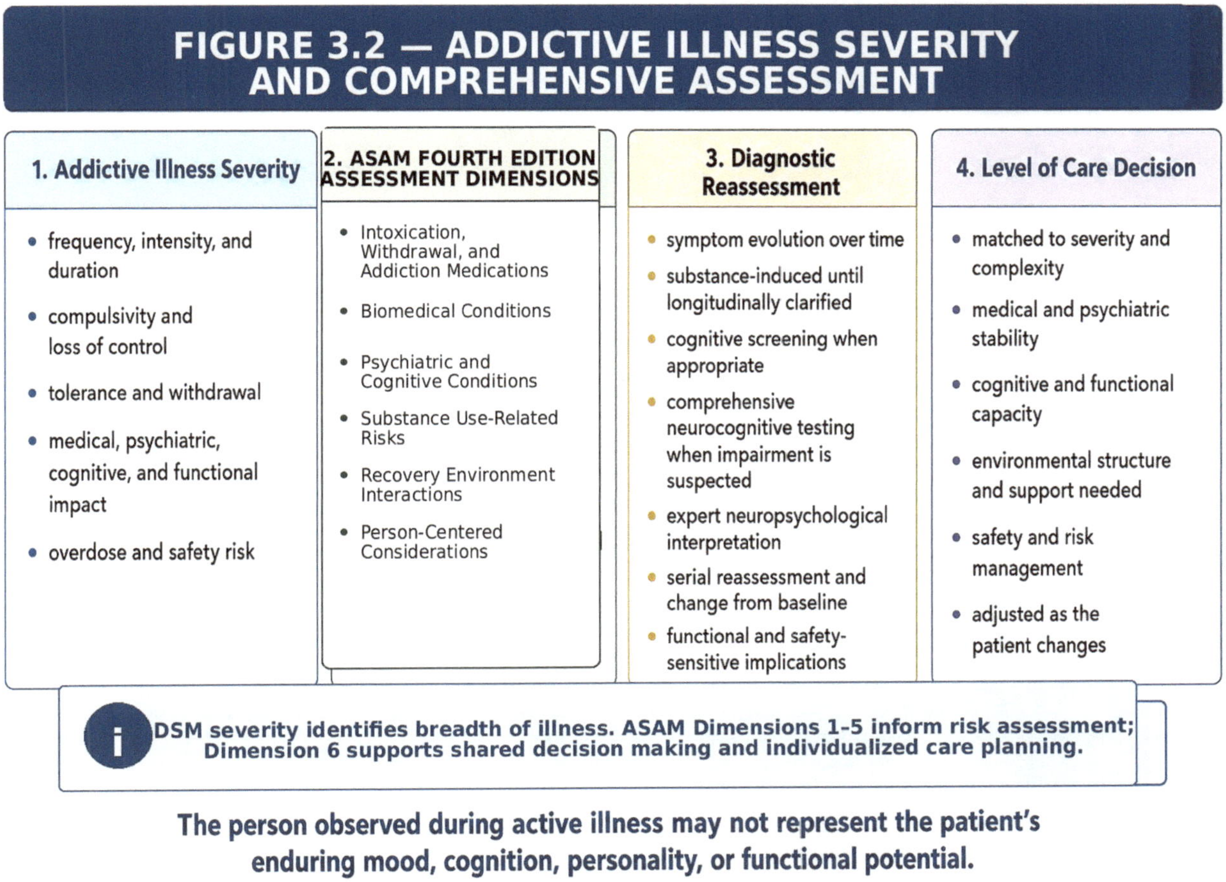

Figure 3.2. Addictive Illness Severity and Comprehensive Assessment. Severity is represented across biological, psychiatric, cognitive, behavioral, functional, environmental, and recurrence-risk domains rather than by substance quantity alone. This figure is a conceptual educational representation, not a validated composite severity scale or level-of-care instrument. Supporting evidence for component mechanisms: [32–33,92].

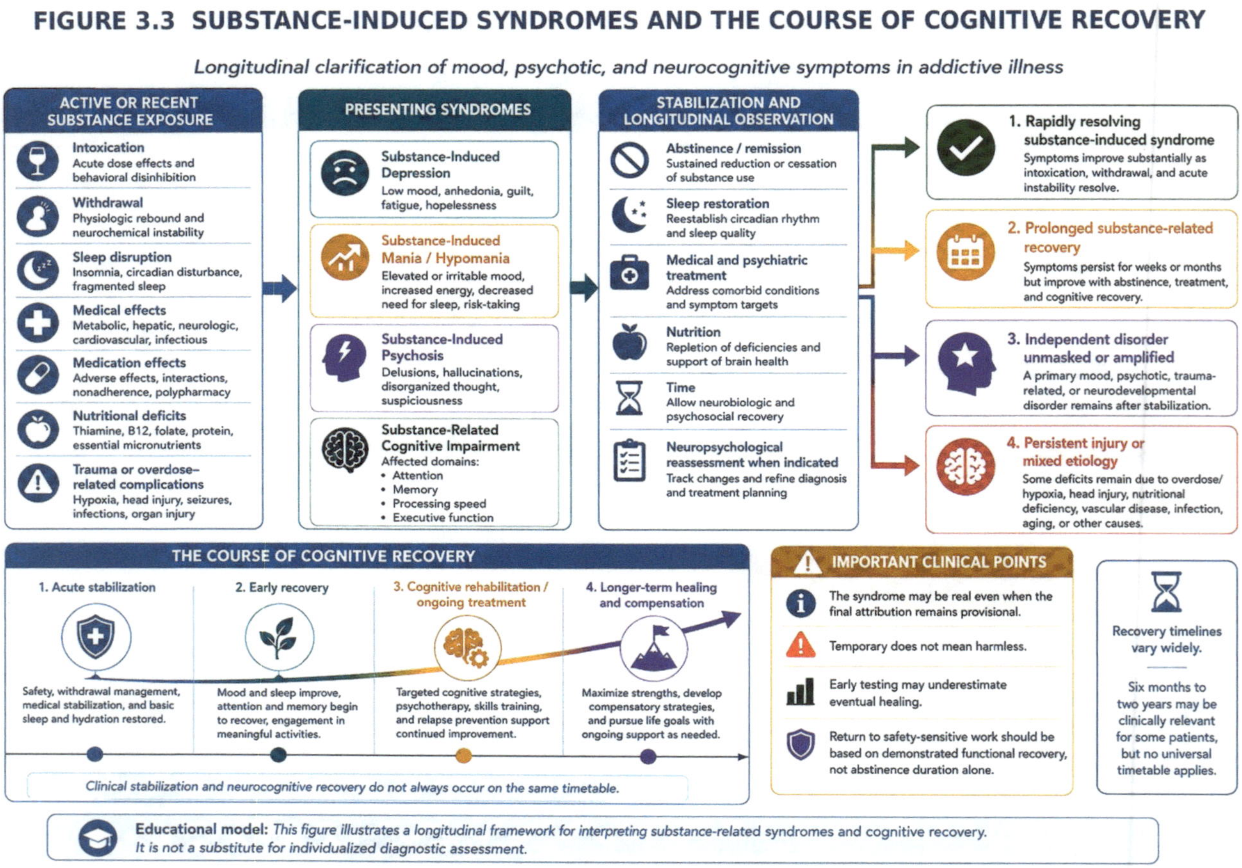

Figure 3.3. Substance-Induced Syndromes and Cognitive Recovery. Serial assessment may help distinguish intoxication, withdrawal, substance-induced syndromes, persistent cognitive effects, and independent psychiatric or neurocognitive disorders. This figure is a conceptual educational representation, not a diagnostic algorithm or universal recovery timeline. Supporting evidence for component mechanisms: [33,47–49].

Personality-Like Behavior During Active Illness

Secrecy, manipulation, emotional volatility, inconsistency, self-centered behavior, reduced empathy, and unstable relationships can appear during severe addictive illness. These behaviors must be taken seriously, and a primary personality disorder may coexist. Clinicians should avoid premature conclusions about enduring personality while the patient remains intoxicated, withdrawing, sleep-deprived, cognitively impaired, acutely traumatized, or otherwise severely dysregulated.

> *Behavior expressed during active illness should be taken seriously without automatically being treated as the patient's enduring personality.*

Longitudinal reassessment after stabilization can clarify whether patterns persist across time and state or substantially improve as the illness is treated. Reassessment complements rather than replaces a warranted diagnostic evaluation.

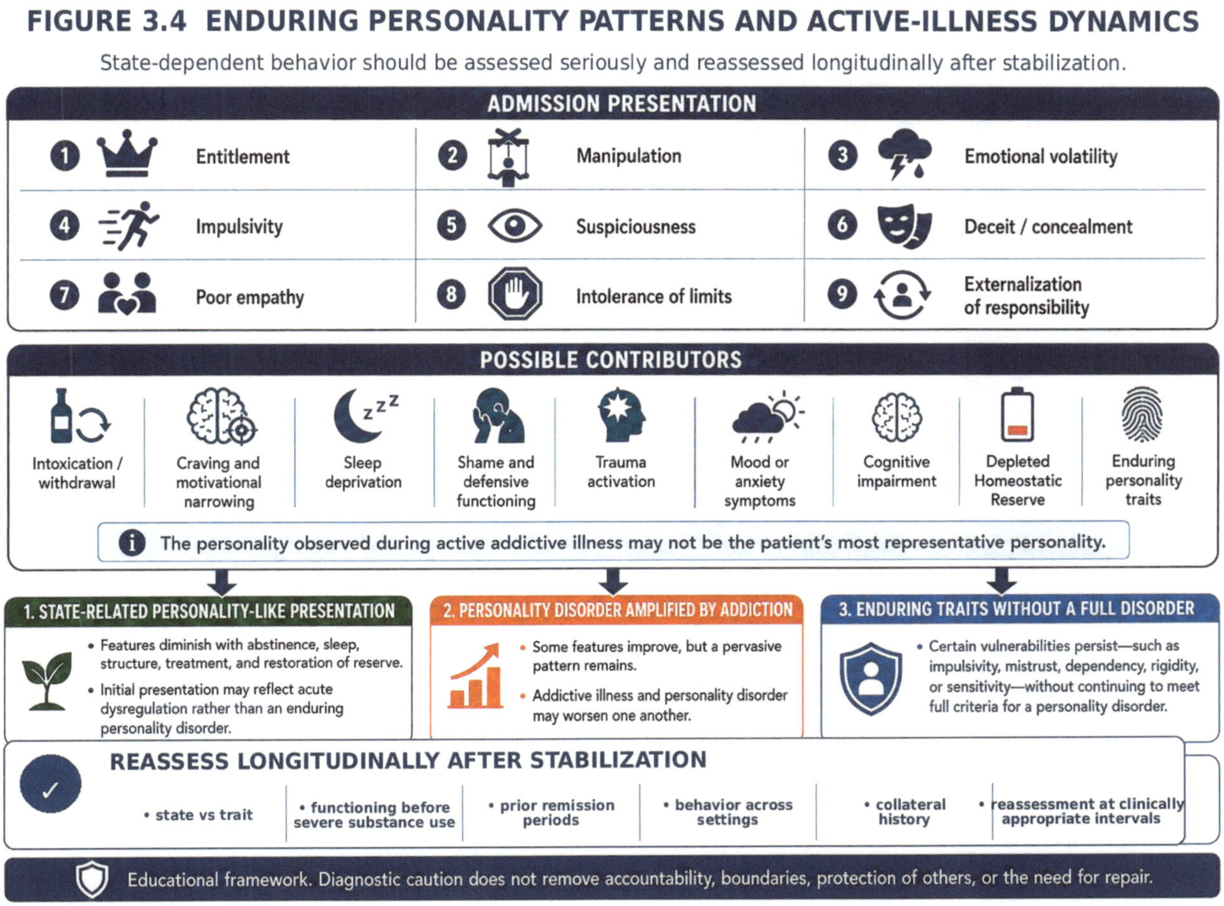

Figure 3.4. Enduring Personality Patterns and Active-Illness Dynamics. Longitudinal reassessment may help distinguish enduring patterns from state-dependent behavior associated with intoxication, withdrawal, sleep loss, trauma activation, cognitive impairment, and depleted reserve. This figure is a conceptual educational representation, not a diagnostic test or rule for deferring diagnosis. Supporting evidence for component mechanisms: [31,33,92].

Selected supporting evidence: [31,33,92].

The Physician's Role

Withdrawal, biomedical illness, psychiatric instability, medication effects, cognitive impairment, and interactions among these domains may require physician involvement. The physician's role is not limited to detoxification; depending on patient need and setting, it may include diagnosis, stabilization, addiction medication, treatment of co-occurring conditions, safety assessment, coordination, and longitudinal interpretation.

Medication may be appropriate while the final diagnostic formulation remains provisional. Treating withdrawal, opioid use disorder, alcohol use disorder, insomnia, depression, anxiety, psychosis, mood instability, pain, or other indicated conditions may improve safety and engagement enough to support more accurate diagnosis and psychotherapy. Medication selection should follow condition-specific evidence and monitoring.

Medication can reduce biological noise enough for the patient to participate in diagnosis and treatment.

Selected supporting evidence: [32,36–37,94].

Recovery-Compatible Medication Principles

Medication choice should begin with the evidence-based indication and an individualized benefit-risk assessment. Onset, route, peak concentration, subjective effects, duration, rebound, misuse potential, diversion risk, interactions, and the patient's learning history may also matter. A slower onset and steadier effect can reduce reinforcement liability for some medications and patients, but this is a heuristic rather than a universal rule.

Rapid-onset and short-duration effects can be more reinforcing in some contexts, but half-life alone does not determine efficacy, safety, misuse risk, or recovery compatibility. Indication-specific evidence, formulation, route, dose, pharmacodynamics, patient history, and available alternatives take precedence over any simple fast-on/fast-off versus slow-on/slow-off distinction.

Selected supporting evidence: [36–46].

Safety-Sensitive Professionals

Physicians, pilots, air-traffic controllers, commercial drivers, transportation workers, public-safety personnel, and others in safety-sensitive roles require an occupation-specific assessment of cognition, judgment, stability, access to substances, monitoring, treatment adherence, functional demand, and public risk under applicable regulatory, licensing, employer, professional-health-program, and specialty standards.

Clinical improvement, conceptual movement above the threshold, or discharge from a level of treatment does not automatically establish fitness for unrestricted duty. Treatment level, remission status, and occupational fitness are related but separate determinations.

Treatment level and fitness for duty are related, but they are not the same determination.

The duty to the patient and the duty to the public are aligned when return is based on demonstrated safety and function.

Selected supporting evidence: [75–80].

Autonomy and Medical Necessity

The patient has the right to accept or refuse recommended care. That right does not require a clinician to certify a clinically inadequate plan as equivalent to the recommended level. When the recommended level is declined, bridge, harm-reduction, or lower-intensity care may be offered when clinically and ethically responsible; it may reduce harm while still being insufficient for the risks identified. The clinician should document the recommendation, alternatives, informed refusal, safety planning, and conditions requiring escalation.

Autonomy permits refusal. It does not require the clinician to misrepresent a lower-intensity plan as equally safe or medically sufficient.

Selected supporting evidence: [32,92,94].

Chapter 3 Closing Perspective

> *Evaluation should describe not only what substance was used, but how much freedom, regulation, cognition, health, and safety the illness has taken.*

That synthesis describes the patient's current state. Part II introduces a framework for understanding why functional capacity can vary so markedly across states and why treatment must sometimes provide what the patient cannot yet sustain alone.

Chapter Summary

Comprehensive evaluation requires more than identifying a substance or counting diagnostic criteria. Clinicians must integrate diagnosis, withdrawal and medical risk, psychiatric and cognitive conditions, functioning, environment, readiness, recurrence risk, and the intensity of structure required for safety and treatment engagement.

Key Clinical Takeaways

- DSM diagnosis and ASAM multidimensional assessment are complementary but not interchangeable.
- Withdrawal management is a phase of care, not a complete treatment episode.
- Medication selection should be diagnosis-specific and evidence-based; onset and half-life are clinical considerations, not standalone measures of appropriateness or abuse liability.
- Treatment progress and occupational fitness-for-duty are related but separate determinations in safety-sensitive work.

PART II
THE HOMEOSTATIC RESERVE FRAMEWORK

The central conceptual contribution of this book

Part II formalizes the Homeostatic Reserve Model and then applies the Homeostatic Threshold to the changing availability of healthy choice.

Authorship and Conceptual Framework Statement

The Homeostatic Reserve Model is an original conceptual framework developed by the author to explain how integrated functional capacity changes across addictive illness, treatment, and recovery. Related terms and neighboring concepts have prior uses in medicine, neuroscience, stress physiology, cognitive reserve, allostasis, frailty, and recovery-capital literature. The originality claimed here lies in the definitions, reserve-threshold architecture, named functional zones, clinical propositions, and integrated application to addictive illness and restoration of value-congruent choice.

> *To the author's knowledge, this framework represents a novel conceptual synthesis rather than a claim to have invented each individual word or every scientific concept incorporated within it.*

The model should be presented confidently but with appropriate scientific humility. It is a framework intended to organize observation, teaching, treatment planning, and future research. It is not represented as a validated biological measurement or a replacement for established diagnostic and placement systems.

Selected supporting evidence: [32–33].

Chapter 4 — The Homeostatic Reserve Model

An Original Conceptual Framework for Addictive Illness and Recovery

The Homeostatic Reserve Model is the central conceptual contribution of this book. It was developed to explain a recurring clinical observation: the same person may know what matters, value what matters, and behave thoughtfully in one state, yet become much less able to act according to those same values when stress, illness, withdrawal, sleep loss, psychiatric symptoms, cue exposure, pain, or cumulative depletion intensify.

> *Why can the same person know what matters, value what matters, and still become temporarily unable to act reliably in accordance with what matters?*

Within the model, this question is approached by focusing on changing functional capacity. The framework integrates biological stability, sleep, physical and psychiatric health, reward responsiveness, executive function, emotional regulation, coping, relationships, environmental resources, meaning, purpose, and hope.

Supporting evidence for component mechanisms: [2–5,28,60]. These sources support component mechanisms; the model's integrated relationship remains an original conceptual proposition.

Why Another Conceptual Model Is Needed

Addiction science has produced powerful models of reinforcement, incentive salience, habit, stress, allostasis, executive dysfunction, and recurrence. Clinical medicine has developed useful concepts of physiological reserve, cognitive reserve, resilience, recovery capital, and social determinants of health. Each describes part of the patient's reality.

The clinical problem is that patients do not experience these domains separately. Sleep loss affects mood, pain, attention, impulse control, craving, and relationships. Withdrawal affects physiology, cognition, emotional regulation, and judgment. Trauma activation affects arousal, memory, trust, and relief seeking. Environmental instability can overwhelm biological and psychological gains. A patient may possess substantial external resources while lacking the current capacity to use them.

Within the Homeostatic Reserve Model, these interacting domains are integrated into one clinical language without reducing addictive illness to one neurotransmitter, one psychological trait, one social problem, or a moral failure.

> *The model asks not only what resources exist, but how much functional capacity the patient currently has to use them.*

Selected supporting evidence: [3,11–12,28,60].

Intellectual Lineage and the Distinctive Synthesis

The words homeostasis, reserve, and threshold are not new. Homeostatic reserve has been used in medicine to describe the capacity to withstand physiological stress. Threshold concepts appear across neuroscience, physiology, cognition, and behavioral science. Addiction models have described altered hedonic set points, allostatic change, stress-system recruitment, sensitization, impaired executive control, and narrowing of motivational salience.

To the author's knowledge, the Homeostatic Reserve Model presented here is distinct in its addiction-specific integration of these neighboring concepts. It defines reserve as an integrated functional capacity rather than a purely physiological reserve, a dopamine supply, willpower, or a list of external assets. For explanatory purposes, it treats the Homeostatic Threshold as a relatively stable conceptual boundary across which the relative availability of survival-oriented relief and value-congruent choice changes. It names the functional zones on either side of that boundary and connects them with treatment scaffolding, recovery capital, natural reward, relationships, honesty, meaning, and restored freedom. This provisional originality statement remains subject to formal database, book, dissertation, conference-proceeding, permissions, and legal review.

> *The proposed originality of the framework lies in the definitions, their relationship, the visual architecture, the clinical propositions, and their application to addictive illness and recovery. The Reserve–Threshold–Trajectory architecture is the central original contribution.*

Selected supporting evidence: [2–4,12,28–29,60].

Formal Definitions

Homeostatic Reserve

Within the Homeostatic Reserve Model, Homeostatic Reserve is defined as the dynamic, integrated functional capacity that allows a person to maintain or regain regulation under stress.

It reflects the combined functional influence of biological stability, restorative sleep, physical and psychiatric health, executive function, emotional regulation, natural reward responsiveness, coping, supportive relationships, environmental resources, meaning, purpose, and hope. No single component is the reserve. Reserve is the resulting regulatory margin created by these systems working together.

> *Formally, reserve names the regulatory margin that remains after current demands are taken into account.*

Homeostatic Threshold

Within the model, the Homeostatic Threshold is treated as a relatively stable conceptual boundary below which survival-oriented relief becomes increasingly dominant and above which reflection, relationships, natural reward, support, and value-congruent choice become more reliably available.

> *The threshold is the line. Reserve is what moves.*

The threshold is not a measured biological cutoff, laboratory value, or claim that human functioning changes at one exact biological point. It is an explanatory boundary within the model that describes a clinically meaningful shift in the relative availability of regulation, freedom, and healthy choice.

The Tank Metaphor

The reserve tank is an educational metaphor. Its apparent level does not represent a literal supply of dopamine, another neurotransmitter, willpower, morality, or a directly measurable biological fluid.

> *The tank represents capacity, not dopamine.*

Dopaminergic function contributes to motivation, salience, effort, anticipation, and reinforcement learning. Hedonic tone contributes to reserve. Neither dopamine nor hedonic tone is identical to Homeostatic Reserve.

Selected supporting evidence: [2–5,9].

What Is in the Homeostatic Reserve Tank?

Within the Homeostatic Reserve Model, the level of the tank represents the resulting regulatory margin created by multiple systems working together. For teaching purposes, the contributing systems can be grouped into seven domains: biological and physiologic stability; psychiatric and emotional regulation; cognitive and executive function; motivational and reward functioning; learned self-regulation and coping; relational and environmental support; and meaning, purpose, and hope.

Genetic contribution and genetic resilience are included within biological and physiologic stability, together with sleep and circadian regulation, nutrition and hydration, physical health, pain burden, withdrawal or intoxication, and autonomic stability. The remaining domains describe the person's emotional and cognitive regulation, responsiveness to natural reward, learned recovery capacities, access to safe relationships and environmental structure, and ability to organize behavior around values and longer-term meaning.

> *These are not separate ingredients poured into the tank. Their interaction determines the person's currently available capacity to regulate, adapt, recover, use support, and act according to values.*

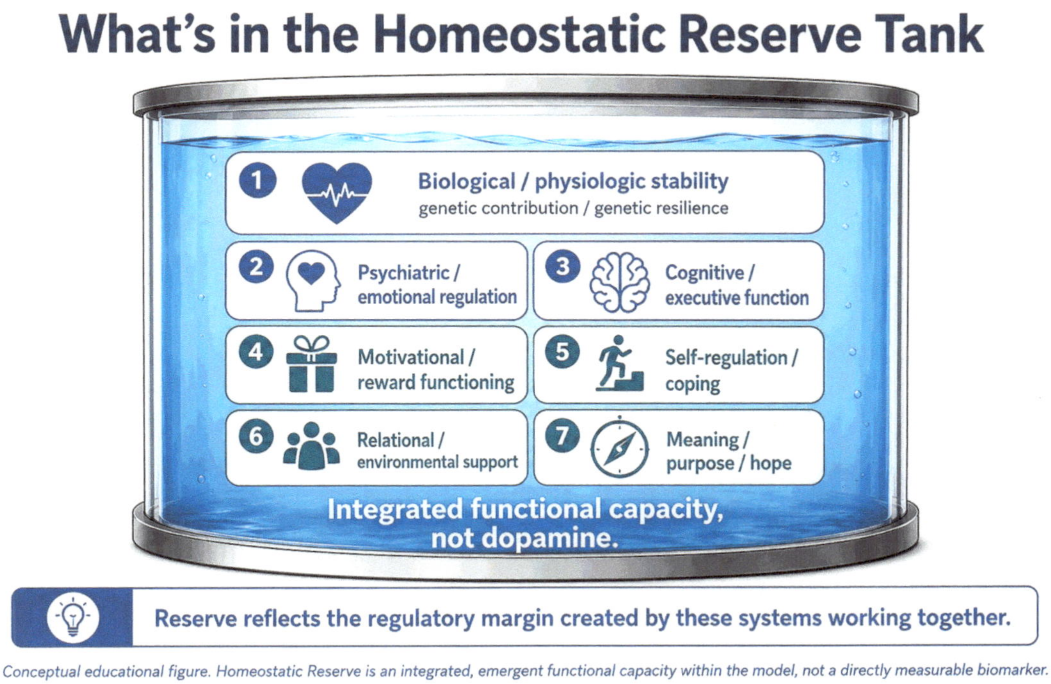

Figure 4.1. What's in the Homeostatic Reserve Tank. Within the model, the tank represents integrated functional capacity produced by interacting biological and physiologic stability, psychiatric and emotional regulation, cognitive and executive function, motivational and reward functioning, learned self-regulation and coping, relational and environmental support, and meaning, purpose, and hope. Genetic contribution and genetic resilience are included within the biological domain. These domains are contributors to reserve, not separate measurable ingredients or a literal dopamine supply. Conceptual educational figure; component mechanisms are supported by [1–5,9–11,13–14,20–22,26,51,60].

Selected supporting evidence: [1–5,9–11,13–14,20–22,26,51,60].

Clinically, the domains can be introduced in sequence without implying a hierarchy. Biological, emotional, and executive systems provide foundational stability; motivational and learned-regulation systems influence how available capacity is used; and relationships, environment, meaning, and hope help sustain and direct that capacity over time.

The Core Architecture of the Model

The model has four central components:

1. A dynamic reserve level representing integrated functional capacity.
2. A Homeostatic Threshold that the model treats, for explanatory purposes, as a relatively stable conceptual boundary.
3. A Survival-Oriented Vulnerability Zone below the threshold.
4. A Value-Congruent Regulatory Zone above the threshold.

Reserve moves as demands and restorative influences change. The same patient may move toward the threshold during grief, illness, sleep loss, conflict, pain, cue exposure, psychiatric destabilization, or withdrawal and move away from it through treatment, sleep, medication, relationships, recovery practice, natural reward, health, meaning, and time.

Within the model, movement across the threshold does not create a different person. It conceptualizes a change in which capacities are most available to the same person in that state.

Selected supporting evidence: [10–11,19,60].

Core Propositions of the Homeostatic Reserve Model

Proposition 1 — Reserve is integrated

Within the model, Homeostatic Reserve reflects the combined functional influence of multiple biological, psychological, cognitive, relational, environmental, and meaning-based systems. It cannot be reduced to one transmitter, receptor, diagnosis, symptom scale, or social resource.

Proposition 2 — Reserve is dynamic

Within the model, reserve changes across time and circumstance. Stress, withdrawal, illness, sleep loss, pain, psychiatric symptoms, cue exposure, isolation, and conflict may lower it. Treatment, sleep, health, medication, relationships, coping, natural reward, purpose, and recovery-supportive behavior may help rebuild it.

Proposition 3 — Baseline reserve differs among individuals

Within the model, inherited biology, development, attachment, trauma, psychiatric and medical burden, prior learning, relationships, and environment may influence the regulatory margin a person possesses before new demands are encountered. The same exposure can therefore acquire very different meaning in different nervous systems.

Proposition 4 — For explanatory purposes, the model treats the threshold as relatively stable while reserve moves

For explanatory purposes, the model treats the threshold as relatively stable rather than requiring it to rise and fall continuously. The patient's reserve level is conceptualized as moving toward, across, and away from the threshold as demands and restorative influences change.

Proposition 5 — Functional freedom changes across the threshold

Within the model, immediate relief, conditioned motivation, urgency, withdrawal, stress, and survival-oriented behavior become increasingly dominant below the threshold. Above it, executive control, natural reward, relationships, support, reflection, honesty, meaning, and values become more reliably available.

This is a probabilistic shift, not an absolute switch. Healthy capacities can remain present below the threshold, and vulnerability remains present above it.

Proposition 6 — Treatment can temporarily supplement insufficient reserve

Within the model, structure may function as borrowed reserve by supplying routines, monitoring, accountability, access reduction, sleep opportunity, and predictable care. Medication may function as biological scaffolding when an indicated treatment reduces withdrawal, craving, psychiatric symptoms, pain, or autonomic distress. The effects and duration of scaffolding vary by condition, medication, adherence, patient, and setting.

Proposition 7 — Recovery capital and Homeostatic Reserve are related but distinct

Recovery capital is an established construct describing resources available to support recovery. Within the Homeostatic Reserve Model, reserve describes the patient's current capacity to recognize, access, tolerate, organize, and use those resources effectively. This distinction is conceptual and has not yet been operationalized against recovery-capital measures.

> *Recovery capital describes what is available. Homeostatic Reserve describes how much capacity the patient has to use what is available.*

Proposition 8 — Recovery is the progressive restoration of functional capacity and freedom

Abstinence may stop ongoing depletion. Active treatment and recovery may help rebuild the capacity to regulate, connect, experience natural reward, use support, tolerate discomfort, act honestly, and live according to values. Restoration is multidomain, heterogeneous, and not assumed to be uniform or complete.

Proposition 9 — The fairness of the fight changes across the threshold

Within the Homeostatic Reserve Model, fairness does not mean that healthy choices are easy, guaranteed, or free of vulnerability. It describes the relative functional and motivational availability of the capacities required for healthy choice.

Within the model, immediate, conditioned, survival-oriented relief holds a disproportionate advantage below the Homeostatic Threshold. As reserve is conceptualized as rising above the threshold, executive control, emotional tolerance, natural reward, relationships, support, meaning, and values become more reliably available. The fight therefore becomes progressively more fair.

Supporting evidence for component mechanisms: [2,10–11,60,63]. These sources support component mechanisms; the model's integrated relationship remains an original conceptual proposition.

What Fills and Drains Reserve

Sleep, nutrition, physical health, psychiatric stability, medication when indicated, emotional regulation, natural reward, supportive relationships, structure, coping skills, honesty, purpose, hope, and time may increase reserve.

Intoxication, withdrawal, insomnia, pain, illness, trauma activation, cue exposure, conflict, secrecy, isolation, psychiatric instability, environmental chaos, and cumulative stress may reduce it.

Different drains may enter through different systems, but they accumulate in the same vulnerable person.

The model does not require that every factor carry equal weight. A severe withdrawal syndrome may dominate the clinical picture in one patient, while chronic pain, grief, insomnia, depression, or environmental instability may be the major drain in another.

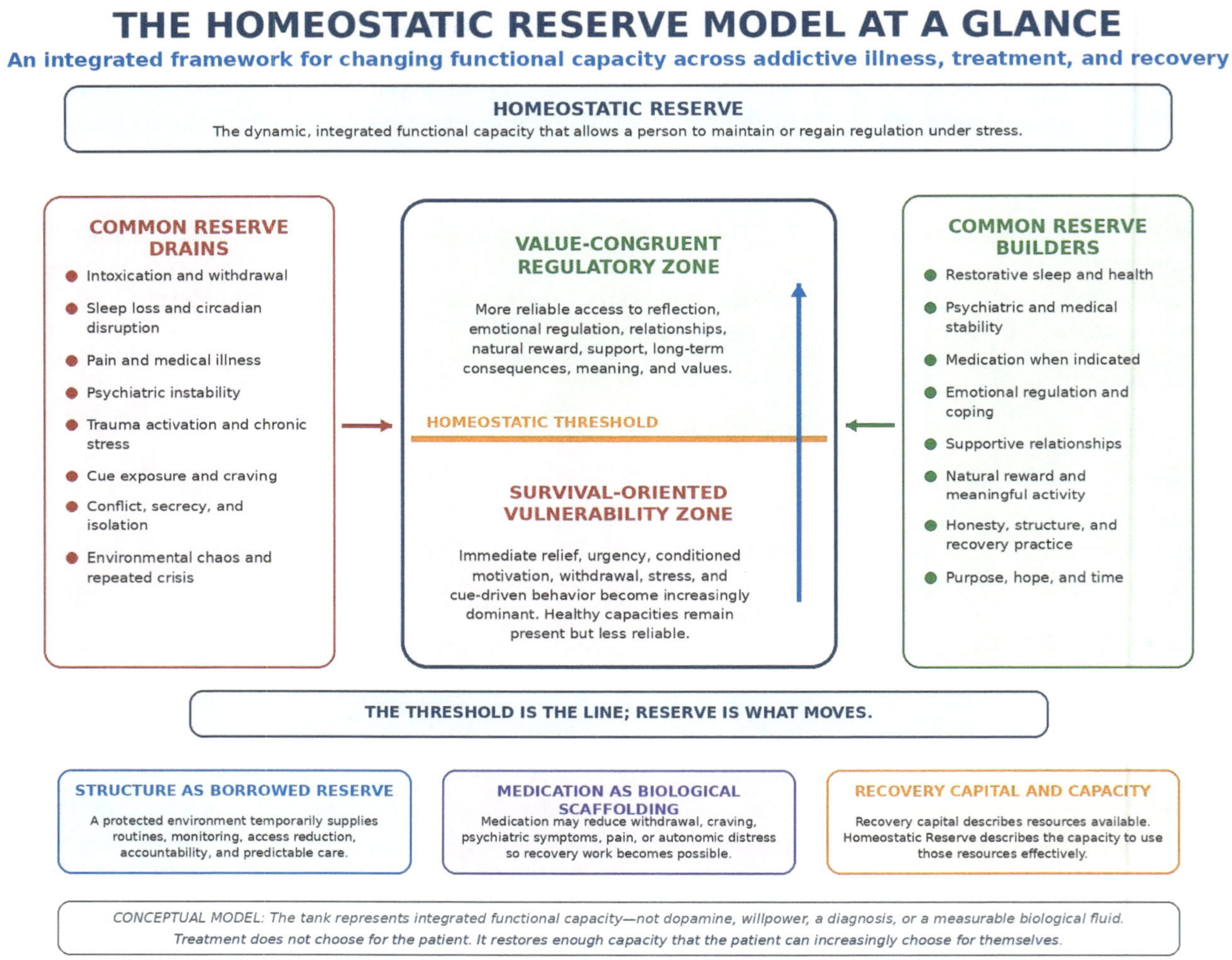

Figure 4.2. The Homeostatic Reserve Model at a Glance. Integrated visual summary of common reserve drains and builders, the Homeostatic Threshold, the Survival-Oriented Vulnerability Zone, the Value-Congruent Regulatory Zone, structure as borrowed reserve, medication as biological scaffolding, and the distinction between recovery capital and the capacity to use it. Within the model, the unfair fight is conceptualized as occurring when depleted reserve lies below the threshold; as reserve rises above it, healthy alternatives become more available and the fight becomes progressively more fair. This figure is a conceptual educational representation, not a validated measurement instrument. The tank represents integrated regulatory capacity, not a literal dopamine or neurotransmitter supply. Supporting evidence for component mechanisms: [2–3,11,28,60].

Selected supporting evidence: [2,20,25,58,60].

Baseline Reserve, Borrowed Normality, and Progressive Depletion

Some people begin life with greater regulatory margin. Others begin closer to the threshold because of inherited biology, development, trauma, psychiatric illness, pain, chronic stress, sleep disruption, or environmental instability.

A substance may initially produce pleasure, relief, or what the model describes as borrowed normality. It may feel as though it provides what the person cannot reliably access: calm, energy, focus, confidence, connection, emotional ease, or sleep. Repeated externally driven regulation may then worsen the baseline it appeared to correct.

> *What begins as an attempt to raise a low baseline may progressively lower the baseline further.*

Selected supporting evidence: [12,21,25,28].

Position Across Recovery

Within the model, the same patient may move from severe depletion through acute stabilization, early recovery, and sustained recovery as reserve rebuilds. Conceptual movement across the threshold increases access to reflection, natural reward, relationships, support, and values, but crossing is not equivalent to a full tank.

Treatment intensity and transitions should follow current authoritative standards, including the ASAM Criteria where applicable, together with individualized clinical judgment and demonstrated function. Within the Homeostatic Reserve Model, reserve offers a conceptual explanation for why apparent improvement within structure may overestimate independent capacity and why step-down should not be based on the passage of time alone.

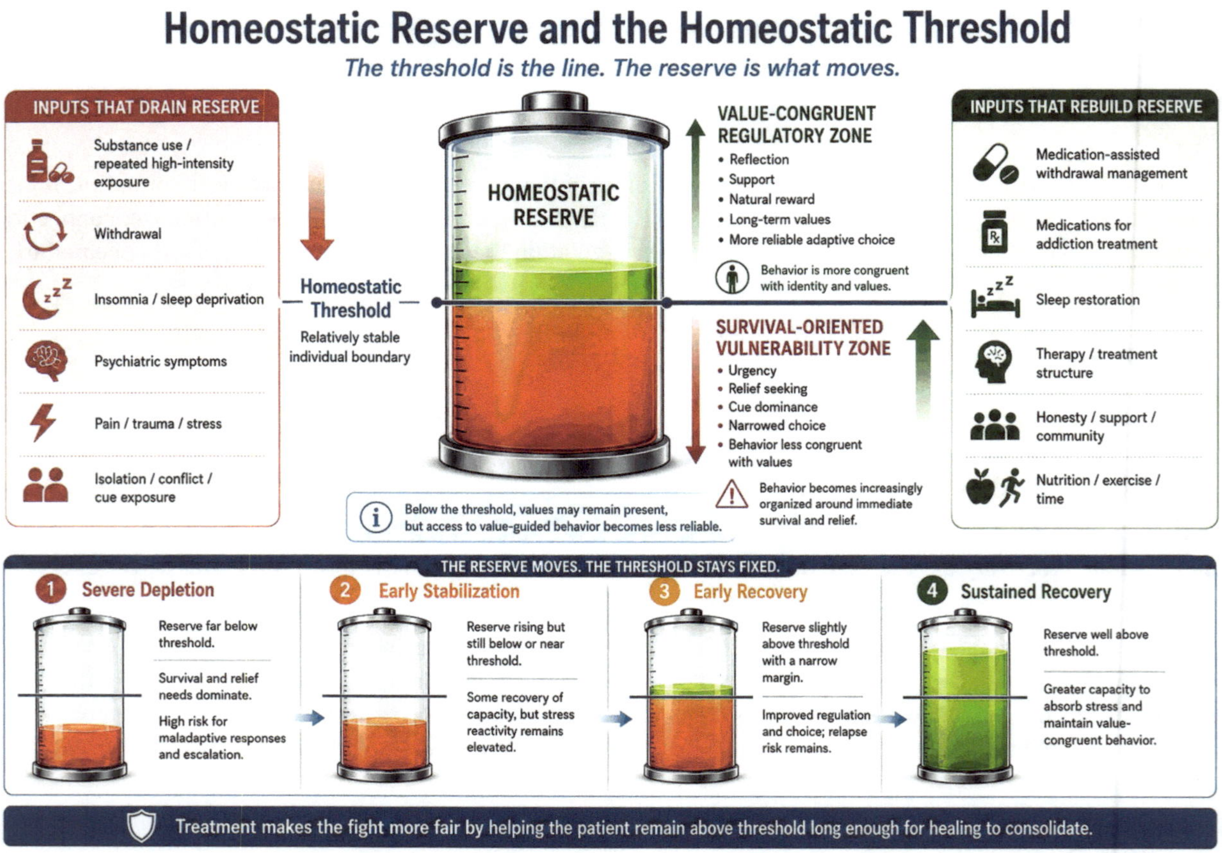

Figure 4.3. Homeostatic Reserve and the Homeostatic Threshold. Within the model, the same patient may move from severe depletion through stabilization and early recovery toward sustained recovery as integrated regulatory capacity rebuilds. Conceptual movement across the threshold increases access to reflection, natural reward, relationships, support, and value-congruent action. This tank-and-threshold figure is a conceptual educational representation, not a validated measurement instrument or measured biological cutoff. The tank represents integrated regulatory capacity, not a literal dopamine or neurotransmitter supply. Supporting evidence for component mechanisms: [52–54].

Supporting evidence for component mechanisms: [52–54,63]. These sources support component mechanisms; the model's integrated relationship remains an original conceptual proposition.

Stress as Cumulative Demand

Stress is broader than subjective anxiety. It includes any biological, psychiatric, medical, relational, cognitive, occupational, or environmental demand that draws on reserve faster than it can be restored.

Stress systems involving the locus coeruleus and norepinephrine, hypothalamic-pituitary-adrenal signaling, corticotropin-releasing factor, dynorphin, and the extended amygdala may intensify negative affect, arousal, craving, and relief seeking. The clinically useful point is not that stress literally empties a dopamine tank, but that stress can increase demand while reward and regulatory systems are already compromised.

Selected supporting evidence: [2,19,25,51].

Structure as Borrowed Reserve and Medication as Biological Scaffolding

When internal capacity is limited, a protected environment can temporarily provide regulation from the outside. Scheduled sleep, meals, medication, therapy, transportation, monitoring, reduced access, accountability, and predictable routines carry functions the patient cannot yet perform reliably.

> *Structure is borrowed reserve.*

Medication may reduce specific biological pressures from withdrawal, craving, psychiatric symptoms, pain, or autonomic distress when it is indicated and effective. Buprenorphine illustrates biological scaffolding in opioid use disorder: it may reduce withdrawal, craving, dysphoria, and preoccupation, stop a major leak, and create a more stable platform from which sleep, relationships, treatment engagement, and recovery behavior can rebuild. These medication effects should not be generalized to every medication or substance-use disorder.

> *Buprenorphine does not fill the entire reserve tank. It may stop a major leak and provide a stable platform from which reserve can rebuild.*

Scaffolding may be temporary, prolonged, or ongoing. Its purpose is health, function, remission, and restored autonomy—not proof that the patient can live without care.

Supporting evidence for component mechanisms: [36–37,39–41]. The Homeostatic Reserve formulation is the author's conceptual synthesis and is not validated by these sources as a composite measure.

From Survival Toward Growth

Maslow's hierarchy provides a useful conceptual parallel rather than a validated recovery staging system. Within the Homeostatic Reserve Model, a patient below the threshold may be organized around immediate biological, emotional, and relational survival. As reserve grows, connection, competence, self-respect, meaning, creativity, and contribution may become more sustainable.

> *Below the threshold, the patient is often trying to survive the internal state. Above the threshold, the patient becomes increasingly able to build a meaningful life.*

This is not a rigid staircase. Love, creativity, spirituality, and meaning can occur during adversity. The claim is narrower: these capacities become easier to sustain when basic regulation and safety are more secure.

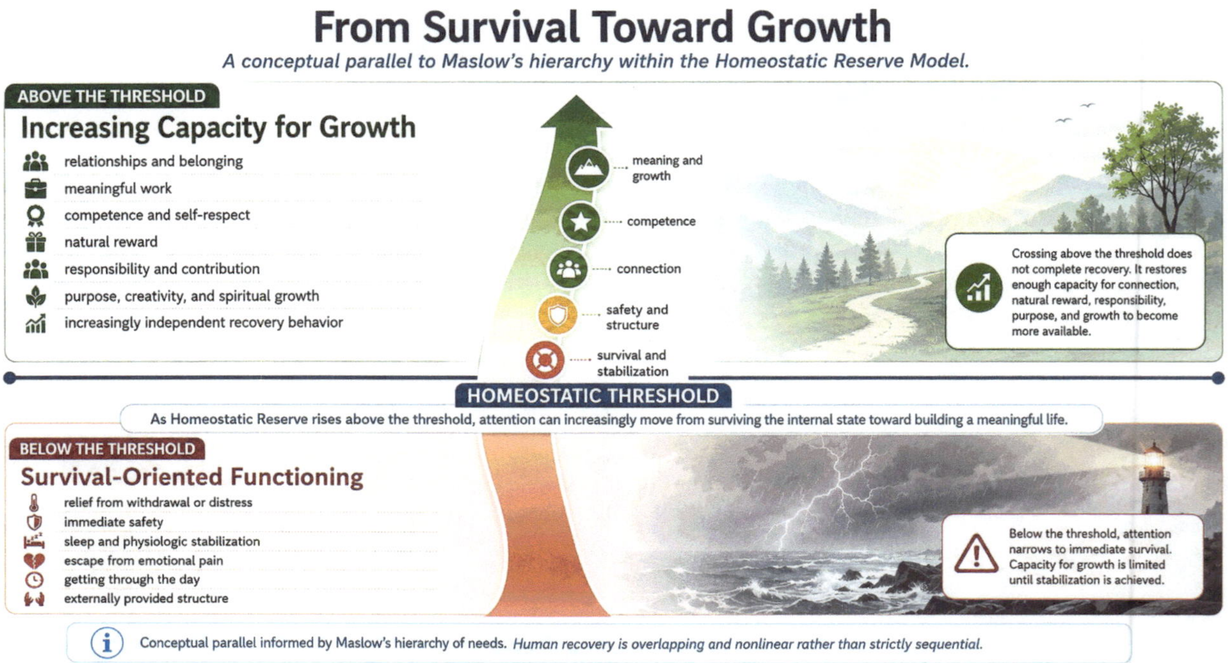

Figure 4.4. From Survival Toward Growth. Conceptual educational parallel integrating Maslow's hierarchy with the Homeostatic Reserve Model. Recovery is overlapping and nonlinear; higher-order experiences may occur during adversity but may be easier to sustain as safety and regulation improve. This figure is not a validated staging or measurement instrument. Supporting evidence for component mechanisms: [58,82–83].

Selected supporting evidence: [57–58,82–83].

What the Model Is—and Is Not

The Homeostatic Reserve Model is:

• a conceptual and educational framework;
• a method for integrating biological, psychiatric, cognitive, relational, and environmental domains;
• a way of understanding changing functional capacity;
• a language for explaining diminished freedom without reducing the patient to morality or one neurotransmitter;
• and a framework for matching treatment support to current vulnerability.

The Homeostatic Reserve Model is not:

• a biomarker or directly measurable biological quantity;
• a literal dopamine tank;
• a DSM diagnosis or ASAM dimension;
• a numerical placement instrument;
• a validated recurrence calculator;
• a fixed statement about personality;
• or a declaration that the patient has no agency or responsibility.

> *Within the model, diminished reserve does not remove responsibility. It proposes why the capacity to carry responsibility may become less reliable in particular states—and why treatment may be necessary to restore it.*

Selected supporting evidence: [32–33,61].

Clinical Questions Generated by the Model

- What is currently draining the patient's reserve?
- What previously provided stable regulation, natural reward, connection, and meaning?
- How close does the patient appear to be to survival-oriented vulnerability?
- Which capacities become unreliable when stress, craving, withdrawal, or sleep loss intensify?
- What must treatment temporarily provide from the outside?
- What biological pressures can medication reduce?
- What recovery capital exists, and can the patient currently use it?
- What evidence would demonstrate that reserve has become sufficiently durable for less structure?

Selected supporting evidence: [3,13,61–62].

Chapter 4 Closing Perspective

> *Within the model, addictive illness is understood as a state in which values may remain intact while the capacity to act on them becomes less reliable.*

Chapter 5 applies this architecture to the functional boundary between survival-oriented vulnerability and value-congruent regulation.

Chapter Summary

The Homeostatic Reserve Model integrates biological, psychiatric, cognitive, motivational, relational, environmental, and meaning-based influences into a single conceptual language for changing functional capacity. Its central contribution is the Reserve–Threshold–Trajectory architecture and its clinical application to addictive illness and recovery.

Key Clinical Takeaways

- Homeostatic Reserve is the resulting regulatory margin created by interacting systems; the seven domains are contributors, not separate substances inside the tank.
- The model treats the threshold as relatively stable for teaching purposes while reserve moves.
- Structure may function as borrowed reserve, and medication may function as biological scaffolding, depending on the patient and condition.
- The model is hypothesis-generating and educational; it is not a validated measurement instrument.

Chapter 5 — The Homeostatic Threshold

From Survival-Oriented Vulnerability to Value-Congruent Choice

Chapter 4 defined the Homeostatic Reserve Model. This chapter applies it clinically. Within the model, the Homeostatic Threshold is treated as a relatively stable conceptual boundary across which the relative availability of immediate relief and value-congruent choice changes. It is not a measured biological cutoff.

> *Crossing the threshold restores possibilities. It does not establish complete recovery.*

Supporting evidence for component mechanisms: [10–11,19]. These sources support component mechanisms; the model's integrated relationship remains an original conceptual proposition.

The Two Functional Zones

The Survival-Oriented Vulnerability Zone

Below the threshold, urgency, withdrawal, craving, cue reactivity, relief seeking, emotional intolerance, cognitive rigidity, isolation, and resistance to help may increase. The nervous system becomes increasingly organized around reducing immediate distress or obtaining the substance that has become the dominant regulator.

Values do not disappear. The patient may continue to love family, care about health, understand consequences, and wish to stop. The problem is that those values become less able to organize behavior in the activated state.

> *Below the threshold, the patient may know what matters while having less reliable access to the capacity required to act on it.*

The Value-Congruent Regulatory Zone

Above the threshold, reflection, emotional regulation, natural reward, relationships, support, honesty, cognitive flexibility, long-term consequences, meaning, and values become more reliably available. The patient is not perfect, fully healed, or invulnerable. The field of choice is broader.

> *Above the threshold, values become more available as guides for behavior rather than only as sources of regret after behavior has occurred.*

Selected supporting evidence: [11,19,51].

How the Fight Changes Across the Threshold

Within the Homeostatic Reserve Model, the threshold marks a clinically meaningful conceptual change in the relative availability and reliability of the capacities required for healthy choice.

Fairness in this context refers to functional availability, not moral deservingness or the theoretical existence of alternatives.

Below the line, immediate relief holds a disproportionate advantage. Near the line, healthier options re-enter the field but remain fragile. With greater margin, those options become more reliable under stress.

The Unfair Fight Proposition

Within the Homeostatic Reserve Model, the Unfair Fight Proposition conceptualizes what may occur when reserve falls below the Homeostatic Threshold: substance-related relief becomes disproportionately immediate, salient, conditioned, and compelling, while healthy alternatives become less motivationally accessible and require regulatory capacity that is currently diminished. This imbalance is the unfair fight of active addictive illness within the model; it is not a measured correlation or biological cutoff.

Treatment alters this imbalance by reducing acute pressures and restoring the capacities that healthy alternatives require.

> *Crossing the threshold does not guarantee healthy choice, and remaining below it does not eliminate all agency. The threshold describes a change in the relative accessibility and reliability of the capacities required for healthy choice.*

Selected supporting evidence: [11–12,19,51].

Adaptive Physiologic Survival and Severe Addictive Illness

The threshold framework can be clarified by comparing severe addictive illness with physiologic survival states without equating them. During starvation or extreme thirst, true physiological deprivation narrows attention and behavior toward food or water. This narrowing is adaptive because restoration of nutrition or hydration directly addresses the underlying deficit.

Severe addictive illness can produce a superficially similar narrowing toward immediate substance-related relief, but through different mechanisms: withdrawal, craving, cue reactivity, stress-system recruitment, reinforcement learning, and less reliable executive control. The substance has acquired survival-like motivational priority even though obtaining it may worsen the underlying illness.

> *Shared principle: when reserve falls below the threshold, behavior narrows toward immediate survival-oriented relief. Key difference: starvation and extreme thirst reflect adaptive physiological deprivation; severe addictive illness reflects a maladaptive, learned survival-like state.*

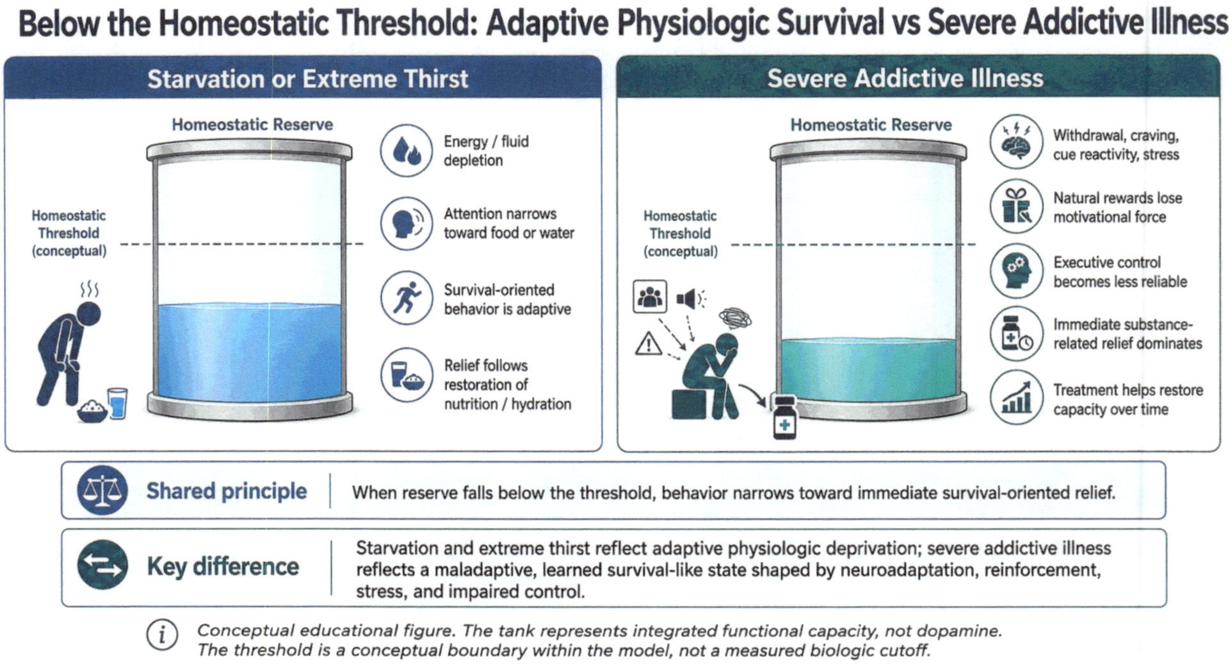

Figure 5.1. Below the Homeostatic Threshold: Adaptive Physiologic Survival Versus Severe Addictive Illness. Starvation and extreme thirst narrow attention and behavior toward restoration of essential physiologic needs. Severe addictive illness may also narrow behavior toward immediate relief, but through withdrawal, craving, conditioned cue reactivity, stress-system recruitment, reinforcement learning, and diminished reliability of executive control. The analogy illustrates behavioral narrowing without claiming that physiological deprivation and addiction are biologically identical. Conceptual educational figure; component mechanisms are supported by [10–12,19,28–29,51,95–96].

Selected supporting evidence: [10–12,19,28–29,51,95–96].

The comparison is therefore explanatory rather than diagnostic. It helps account for why a patient may sincerely want to stop while immediate relief continues to dominate behavior, and why treatment must reduce the underlying pressures rather than rely on information or willpower alone.

The Zones Are Probabilistic, Not Absolute

The model does not claim that every person below the threshold behaves identically or that every person above it makes healthy decisions. It describes a shift in probability and reliability.

A patient below the threshold may still ask for help, tell the truth, refuse a substance, or protect another person. A patient above the threshold may still make an impulsive or unhealthy decision. The clinically important change is how available and repeatable healthier capacities become under stress.

> *The threshold describes a change in the reliability of capacity, not the presence or absence of human worth.*

Selected supporting evidence: [2,19,53].

Crossing the Threshold Is Not a Full Tank

A patient may move just above the threshold and regain enough capacity to participate, accept medication, disclose risk, ask for help, or make a safer decision while remaining highly vulnerable. Greater distance above the threshold provides more margin for illness, conflict, cue exposure, disappointment, pain, sleep loss, and ordinary life demands.

> *Just above the threshold is clinically better, but it is not the same as well above the threshold.*

A patient may look dramatically improved within a highly structured setting because the environment is carrying much of the regulatory burden. The question is not only whether the patient looks better, but how much of that improvement can be sustained as external support decreases.

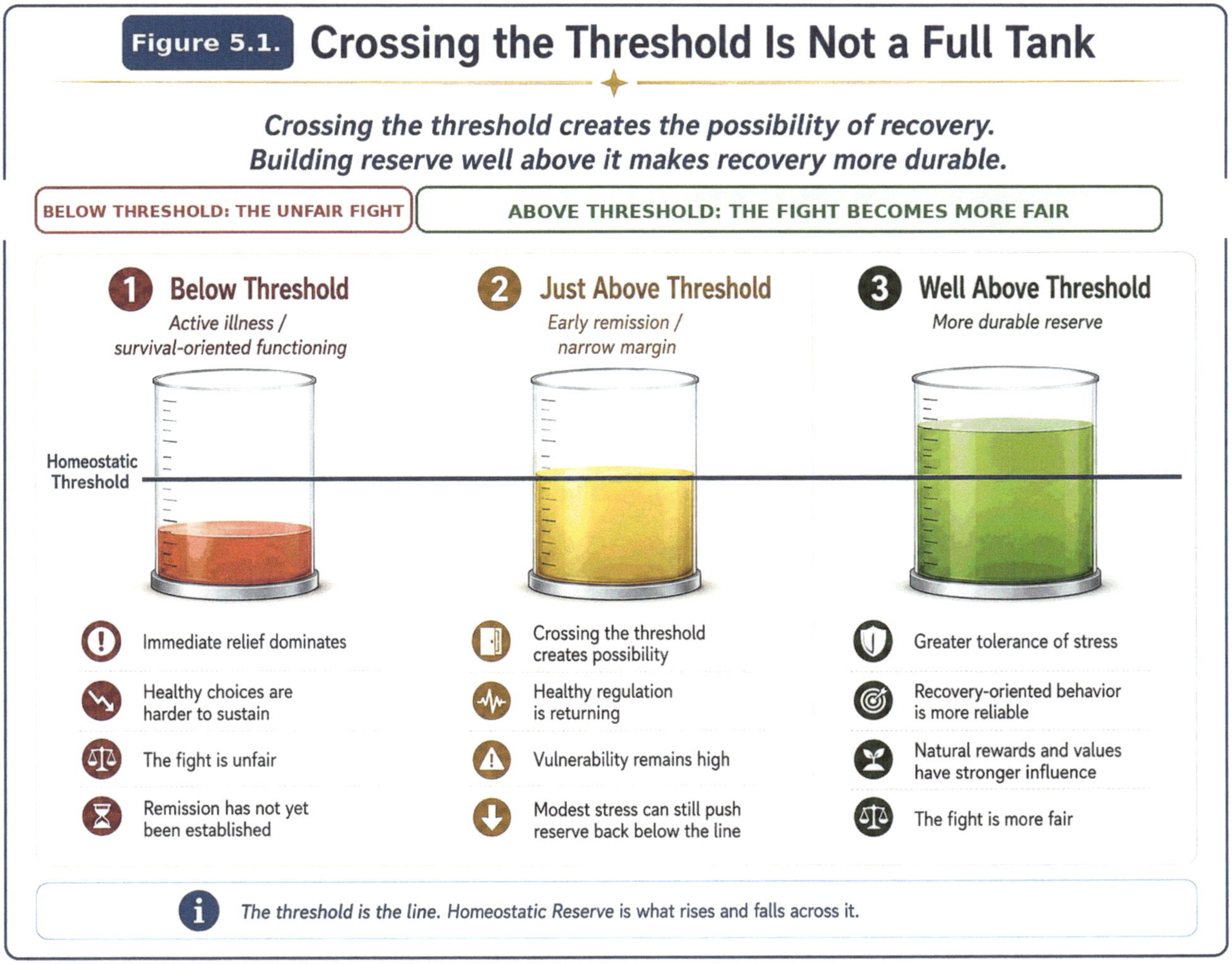

Figure 5.2. Crossing the Threshold Is Not a Full Tank. Within the model, the area below the threshold represents the unfair fight: survival-oriented relief holds a disproportionate advantage and healthy choices are harder to sustain. Just above the threshold, the fight becomes more fair but remains fragile. Well above the threshold, healthier alternatives become more reliably available and the fight becomes increasingly more fair and durable. This tank, threshold, and zone figure is a conceptual educational representation, not a validated measurement instrument or measured biological cutoff. The tank represents integrated regulatory capacity, not a literal dopamine or neurotransmitter supply. Supporting evidence for component mechanisms: [11,19,51].

Selected supporting evidence: [52–54].

How Treatment Makes the Fight More Fair

Within the model, a patient below the threshold is not choosing between equally available alternatives. The substance-related option may offer immediate relief, certainty, familiarity, intense reinforcement, and strongly conditioned behavioral pathways. The healthy alternative may offer delayed benefit, uncertainty, effort, emotional discomfort, and little immediate reward. This is the clinical expression of the Unfair Fight Proposition.

> *Within the Homeostatic Reserve Model, active addictive illness creates an unfair fight between immediate survival-oriented relief and healthy behavior whose benefits are slower, less certain, and harder for the patient to feel.*

Treatment changes the conditions of the fight. It may reduce biological pressure, create time, limit access, supply relationships, restore sleep, build skills, and allow natural reward and long-term values to regain motivational force. As reserve is conceptualized as crossing and continuing to rise above the threshold, healthy alternatives become more genuinely available and increasingly durable.

> *Treatment makes the fight more fair—not by choosing for the patient, but by restoring enough capacity that healthy choice can compete more effectively.*

Selected supporting evidence: [36–37,39,63,65].

Recovery-Oriented Action Can Begin Below the Threshold

Patients do not need perfect insight or complete internal motivation before treatment begins. Entering treatment, accepting medication, following structure, telling part of the truth, attending group, allowing collateral information, or accepting a family boundary may begin filling the tank before stable remission is established.

> *Action can begin before complete insight, and treatment can create the conditions in which insight grows.*

This principle protects against a common error: withholding adequate treatment until the depleted patient demonstrates the very capacities treatment is intended to restore.

Selected supporting evidence: [63,66,69].

Failure to Establish Remission Versus Recurrence After Remission

Within this framework, a patient who continues using, repeatedly returns to use during early stabilization, or never develops enough protection to establish remission may be more accurately described as having persistent active illness or failure to establish remission rather than recurrence after remission.

Within this framework, recurrence refers to renewed illness activity after a meaningful period of established remission or recovery. Reserve may fall as sleep deteriorates, psychiatric illness returns, stress accumulates, honesty decreases, treatment participation declines, cue exposure intensifies, medication is stopped, support weakens, or recovery capital changes.

This is a clinically useful distinction within the Homeostatic Reserve framework, not a new DSM or ASAM diagnostic category. Failure to establish remission suggests that treatment intensity, breadth, duration, engagement, or fit may have been insufficient for the risks present. Recurrence after remission warrants reassessment of how a previously protective recovery system was weakened, exceeded, or no longer matched to the conditions that developed.

Persistent active illness and recurrence after remission require related but different clinical explanations.

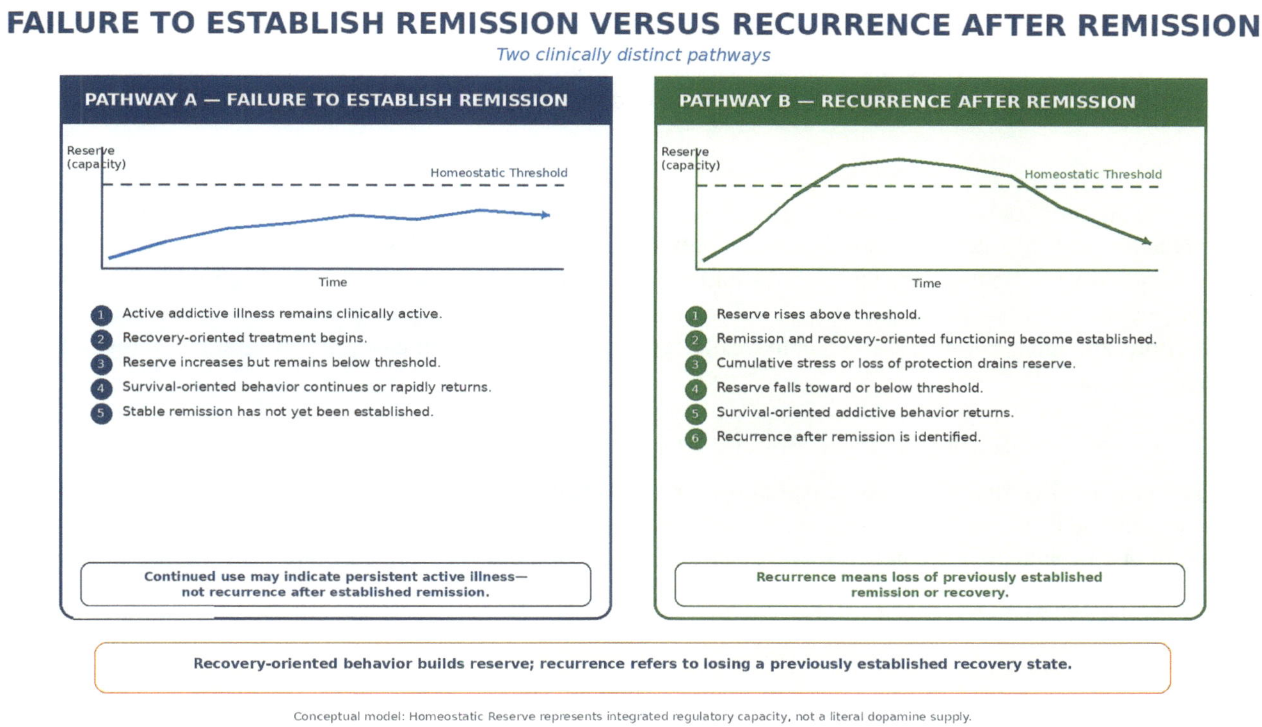

Figure 5.3. Failure to Establish Remission Versus Recurrence After Remission. One conceptual pathway represents persistent active illness without stable remission. The other represents established recovery followed by declining reserve and renewed illness activity. This is a clinically useful distinction within the framework, not a formal DSM or ASAM taxonomy. The figure is a conceptual educational representation, not a validated measurement or recurrence-prediction instrument. The tank represents integrated regulatory capacity, not a literal dopamine or neurotransmitter supply. Supporting evidence for component mechanisms: [33,63,91].

Selected supporting evidence: [33,63,91].

Structured Treatment Can Make the Illness More Visible

Structured treatment can remove intoxication and access, observe behavior over time, integrate medical and psychiatric data, gather collateral information within appropriate consent, confidentiality, and legal boundaries, and allow patients to recognize themselves in the stories of others.

Structured treatment can make the illness more visible.

The patient may move from viewing several consequences as separate accidents toward recognizing one powerful illness requiring a treatment plan strong enough to match it. Structure also reveals whether improvement reflects internalized recovery or continued dependence on external regulation.

Selected supporting evidence: [32,65,69].

Clinical Applications of the Threshold Model

Severe withdrawal and sleep loss

A patient in withdrawal who has slept little for several nights may understand the medical risks and still become unable to tolerate the immediate state. Medication-assisted withdrawal management during the detoxification phase, restorative sleep, and structured care may reduce acute pressures and, within the model, help raise reserve enough for treatment participation and safer decision-making.

A safety-sensitive professional

A physician, pilot, or other safety-sensitive professional may be articulate, knowledgeable, and highly motivated while still showing state-dependent deficits in judgment, attention, self-monitoring, or stress tolerance. Improvement or conceptual threshold crossing within treatment does not by itself establish fitness for duty. Occupational readiness is a separate determination that requires durable function under realistic conditions and must follow the applicable regulatory, licensing, professional-health-program, employer, and specialty standards.

High recovery capital but limited capacity to use it

A patient may have financial resources, family support, excellent clinicians, transportation, and stable housing yet remain unable to use those resources consistently because depression, insomnia, withdrawal, cognitive impairment, or denial has depleted reserve. The problem is not absence of opportunity. It is limited current capacity to convert opportunity into recovery action.

Medication and structure supporting threshold crossing

A patient with opioid use disorder may remain below the threshold because withdrawal, craving, dysphoria, and preoccupation consume much of the available capacity. Buprenorphine and a structured environment may reduce these drains, allowing sleep, treatment engagement, relationships, honesty, and executive control to become more available. This medication-specific example should not be generalized to every medication or substance-use disorder.

Recognizing decline before recurrence

A patient in stable recovery may begin sleeping poorly, missing meetings, isolating, becoming less honest, romanticizing prior use, or discontinuing medication. Substance use has not yet occurred, but within the model reserve may be falling toward the threshold. Early intervention may restore protection before judgment and freedom narrow further.

Selected supporting evidence: [32,34,36,60,77].

Clinical Use Without False Precision

There is no clinical glucometer for addictive illness. Homeostatic Reserve cannot currently be read as one number, and the Homeostatic Threshold is not a measured biological cutoff and should not be assigned an arbitrary laboratory value.

Clinical assessment instead integrates behavior, trajectory, sleep, cognition, emotional regulation, psychiatric and medical stability, craving, honesty, relationships, use of support, functional performance, collateral information, and response to changing structure.

> *The model is most useful when it improves clinical questions, not when it creates false numerical certainty.*

Selected supporting evidence: [32,61–62].

Potential Domains for Future Measurement

The model can generate testable research questions without claiming current validation. Potential domains include:

- sleep and circadian stability;
- executive function and cognitive flexibility;
- hedonic tone and natural reward responsiveness;
- stress reactivity and emotional regulation;
- craving and cue reactivity;
- psychiatric and medical stability;
- social connection and attachment security;
- honesty and early disclosure of vulnerability;
- treatment participation and recovery behavior;
- functional performance under changing levels of structure;
- and the ability to recognize and use recovery resources.

Future research could examine whether combinations of these domains help predict conceptual threshold crossing, successful step-down, return to function, or recurrence more accurately than any single measure. These are candidate domains for study, not a provisional Homeostatic Reserve score.

Selected supporting evidence: [3,13,58,61–62].

Agency, Responsibility, and Compassion

Within the model, the threshold does not erase agency, excuse harm, or remove accountability. It offers a conceptual description of why agency may become less reliable in particular states and why responsibility may need to be supported through treatment, structure, monitoring, and time.

> *The model does not remove responsibility. It helps match responsibility to actual capacity and treatment to actual need.*

This framing allows compassion and accountability to coexist. The patient is responsible for participating in treatment, disclosing risk, repairing harm, and protecting recovery as capacity returns. Clinicians and families are responsible for not confusing depleted capacity with bad character or expecting independence before the patient can sustain it safely.

Selected supporting evidence: [69,73–74].

Chapter 5 Closing Perspective

> *The threshold marks a change in available capacity, not a declaration that healing is complete.*

The Threshold describes functional position; the Healing Trajectory in Chapter 6 describes how that position changes over time.

Chapter Summary

The Homeostatic Threshold organizes the model into two probabilistic functional zones. Below it, immediate relief and survival-oriented motivation gain disproportionate advantage; above it, reflection, support, natural reward, and value-congruent action become more reliably available.

Key Clinical Takeaways

- Below-threshold states do not erase values, agency, or responsibility; they change the reliability and relative availability of healthy capacities.
- Starvation and extreme thirst provide an analogy for adaptive survival-oriented narrowing, whereas severe addictive illness reflects a maladaptive learned survival-like state.
- Crossing the threshold is not the same as full recovery or a full tank.
- Treatment makes the fight more fair by reducing destabilizing pressures and rebuilding the capacity required for healthy choice.

PART III
TREATMENT, HEALING, AND RECOVERY

Stage-matched treatment, rebuilding reserve, protecting remission, and living beyond survival

Chapter 6 adds time to the model. Chapter 7 explains how multidisciplinary treatment should change as capacity rebuilds. Chapters 8 through 12 then follow recovery from rebuilding and environment, through insight and maintenance, toward meaningful living.

Chapter 6 — The Homeostatic Reserve Healing Trajectory

How Integrated Regulatory Capacity Rebuilds Over Time

Chapters 4 and 5 described Homeostatic Reserve and the patient's conceptual functional position relative to the Homeostatic Threshold. This chapter adds the temporal dimension of the model: how reserve may rebuild, fluctuate, cross the threshold, and become increasingly durable over time.

> *Reserve describes capacity. Threshold describes functional position. Trajectory describes change over time.*

Healing may begin before the patient can feel it. Abstinence may interrupt intoxication, withdrawal, and continued depletion, but sleep, stress regulation, cognition, natural reward, emotional regulation, relationships, insight, and identity recover at different rates.

Supporting evidence for component mechanisms: [52–54,57,63]. These sources support component mechanisms; the model's integrated relationship remains an original conceptual proposition.

Formal Definition

> *Within the Homeostatic Reserve Model, the Homeostatic Reserve Healing Trajectory is conceptualized as the nonlinear, multidomain process through which a person progressively rebuilds the biological, cognitive, emotional, relational, motivational, and meaning-based capacity required to maintain regulation and live according to values.*

The phrase healing trajectory has prior use across medicine, rehabilitation, psychology, and addiction treatment. To the author's knowledge, the distinctive contribution proposed here is not the generic observation that people heal over time. It is the formal integration of time with Homeostatic Reserve, the Homeostatic Threshold, multiple domains of recovery, treatment scaffolding, recovery capital, and restoration of value-congruent choice.

Within the Homeostatic Reserve Model, the Healing Trajectory is the temporal component of the central Reserve–Threshold–Trajectory architecture.

Selected supporting evidence: [52–54,57].

Why a Temporal Model Is Needed

A patient can be abstinent and still have limited capacity. A patient can look significantly improved within structure and remain unable to sustain the same level of functioning independently. One domain can improve while another remains impaired. A temporary setback can lower reserve without erasing every gain that preceded it.

A calendar alone cannot explain these differences. The relevant clinical question is not simply, "How long has the patient been abstinent?" It is also, "What capacities have returned, how reliably are they available, what conditions are supporting them, and how durable are they under stress?"

> *Time creates the opportunity for healing. Comprehensive treatment can help convert that opportunity into restored capacity.*

Selected supporting evidence: [47,52–53,63].

Core Propositions of the Homeostatic Reserve Healing Trajectory

Proposition 1 — Healing is multidomain

Recovery involves more than cessation of substance use. Biological stability, sleep, cognition, executive control, emotional regulation, natural reward, relationships, insight, honesty, recovery identity, meaning, and value-congruent action may all contribute to the rebuilding of reserve.

Proposition 2 — Different domains heal at different rates

Withdrawal may improve before sleep. Sleep may improve before executive function. Cognitive performance may improve before emotional tolerance. Insight may deepen before relationships are repaired. Natural reward and recovery identity may take longer to become durable.

Improvement in one domain does not mean that all capacities have been restored.

Proposition 3 — Healing is nonlinear

Reserve may rise, plateau, fluctuate, or temporarily fall. Illness, grief, insomnia, psychiatric symptoms, pain, cue exposure, conflict, overwork, and environmental instability can consume reserve even after meaningful progress has occurred. Nonlinearity does not mean that recovery is not real.

Proposition 4 — Abstinence may precede restored capacity

The patient may stop using before becoming able to tolerate distress, experience ordinary reward, use support, recognize risk, or make healthy decisions reliably. The absence of intoxication therefore cannot be treated as proof that executive, emotional, motivational, or relational recovery is complete.

The absence of acute intoxication does not establish the presence of restored capacity.

Proposition 5 — Crossing the threshold is a milestone, not an endpoint

Within the model, as reserve rises above the Homeostatic Threshold, reflection, natural reward, relationships, support, honesty, and value-congruent choice become more available. A patient just above the threshold may still have little margin for stress and may remain dependent on structure and treatment support.

Threshold crossing is a milestone in recovery, not evidence that every system has healed.

Proposition 6 — External scaffolding can support the trajectory while capacity internalizes

Structure may function as borrowed reserve, and medication may function as biological scaffolding. The treatment team may temporarily provide regulation, interpretation, monitoring, hope, routine, accountability, and protection until the patient can increasingly perform those functions independently.

Proposition 7 — The trajectory is shaped by both internal capacity and external conditions

Recovery capital, housing, family, work demands, treatment access, community support, substance availability, digital cues, finances, and transportation can accelerate, slow, or destabilize the trajectory. Healing occurs within an environment, not outside it.

Proposition 8 — Treatment transitions should follow demonstrated function, not time alone

Time in care matters because biological and psychological healing require time. Treatment transitions should follow current authoritative criteria and individualized clinical judgment. Within the model, step-down and increasing independence are conceptualized as tests of demonstrated, durable function under increasingly realistic conditions; return to safety-sensitive duties requires a separate occupational-fitness determination under applicable standards.

Supporting evidence for component mechanisms: [52–54,60,63]. These sources support component mechanisms; the model's integrated relationship remains an original conceptual proposition.

Four Broad Heuristic Phases of the Trajectory

Acute stabilization — illustrative guidepost: days to early weeks

The priorities are safety, withdrawal management, sleep opportunity, medical and psychiatric stabilization, nutrition, hydration, reduction of access, and enough regulation for the patient to participate in treatment. Apparent decisiveness during this phase may be unstable and state-dependent.

Early rebuilding — illustrative guidepost: several weeks to approximately three months

The patient begins practicing structure, emotional regulation, recovery behavior, medication adherence, honest disclosure, group participation, and use of support. Sleep, attention, and mood may improve, while reward responsiveness, insight, and independent judgment remain fragile.

Consolidation — illustrative guidepost: approximately three to twelve months

Recovery behaviors become more practiced and less dependent on moment-to-moment prompting. The patient tests capacity under greater responsibility, strengthens relationships, develops recovery identity, and begins addressing deeper psychiatric, relational, trauma, grief, or medical burdens when sufficiently stable.

Integration — illustrative guidepost: one year and beyond

Recovery becomes increasingly integrated into identity, values, relationships, work, service, and ordinary life. Vulnerability remains, but the patient has greater margin, earlier recognition of decline, and more reliable pathways back toward regulation.

These phases and date ranges are heuristic guideposts, not expected biological deadlines, promises, or a universal sequence. Timing differs by substance, duration and intensity of exposure, age, health, comorbidity, treatment, environment, and the recovery domain being considered. A patient may move differently across domains, return temporarily to greater support, or require long-term medication and monitoring without that representing failure.

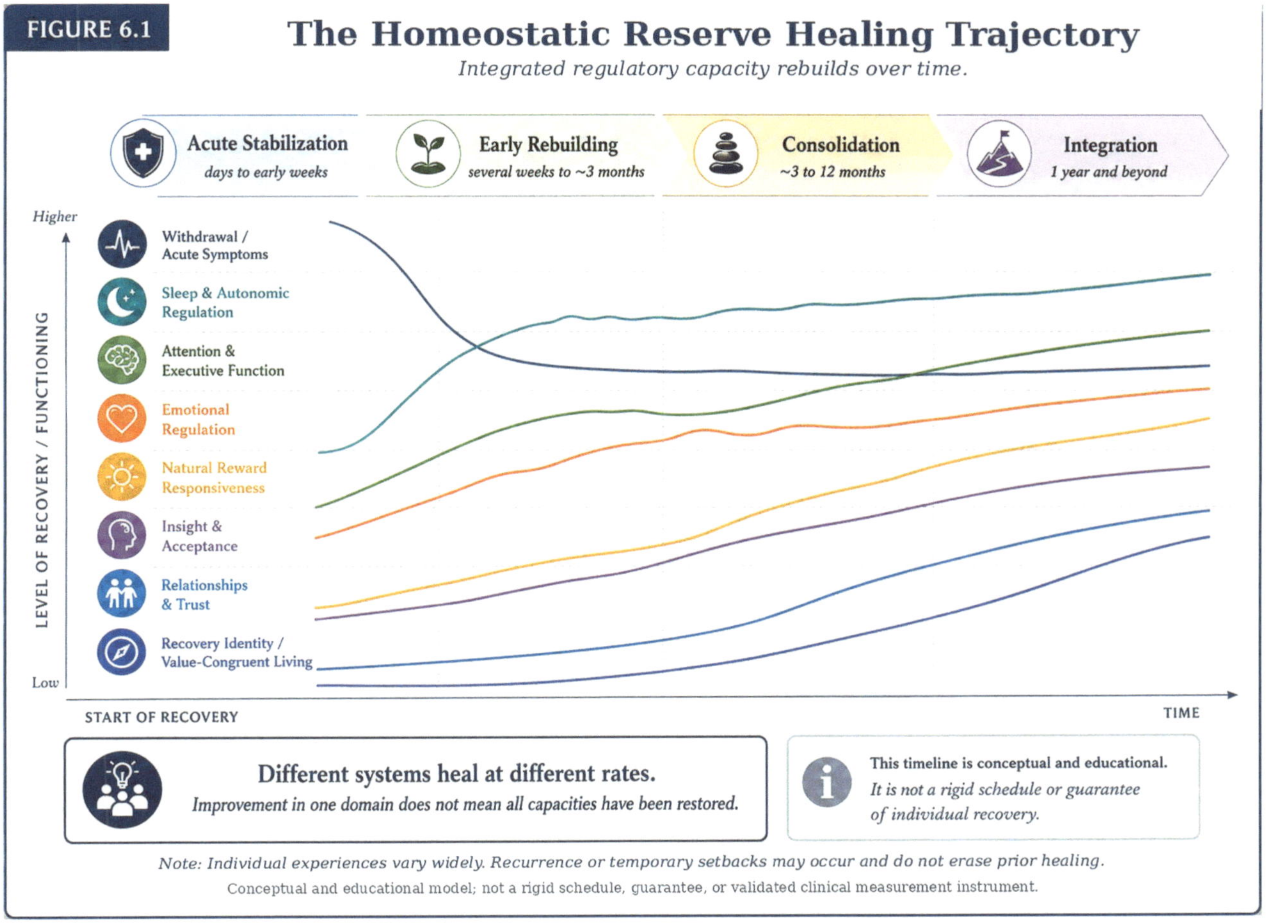

Figure 6.1. The Homeostatic Reserve Healing Trajectory. Conceptual temporal model illustrating that withdrawal and acute symptoms, sleep and autonomic regulation, attention and executive function, emotional regulation, natural reward responsiveness, insight and acceptance, relationships and trust, and recovery identity may change at different rates across heuristic phases of acute stabilization, early rebuilding, consolidation, and integration. All curves and date ranges are illustrative; the withdrawal and acute-symptom curve does not imply that post-acute symptoms persist in every patient or follow one fixed course. This trajectory figure is a conceptual educational representation, not a validated measurement scale or universal schedule. Homeostatic Reserve represents integrated regulatory capacity, not a literal dopamine or neurotransmitter supply. Supporting evidence for component mechanisms: [47,52–55].

Selected supporting evidence: [47,52–54].

Different Systems Heal at Different Rates

Acute withdrawal symptoms may fall rapidly while insomnia, autonomic instability, or dysphoria persist. Attention and executive function may improve gradually. Emotional regulation can fluctuate as the patient begins to experience feelings previously suppressed or avoided. Natural reward may return slowly, requiring the patient to engage in healthy activity before being able to feel its full value.

Insight and acceptance may deepen as cognition improves, shame decreases, and the patient observes the illness across time. Relationships and trust generally require repeated evidence. Recovery identity and value-congruent living become stronger through practice rather than declaration.

The patient may be doing healthy things before the brain has fully recovered the ability to feel their value.

Selected supporting evidence: [47,52–55].

Treatment Must Change as Capacity Changes

The Healing Trajectory explains why treatment that is useful during acute stabilization may differ from treatment that becomes useful after weeks or months of rebuilding. Early care may need to be more concrete, protective, repetitive, and externally structured; later care may become more direct, exploratory, and focused on responsibility, grief, trauma, relationships, identity, and meaning. Chapter 7 develops this stage-matched multidisciplinary treatment approach in detail.

The trajectory describes changing capacity. Effective treatment changes with it.

Selected supporting evidence: [32,63,69,71–72,92,94].

Nonlinearity, Temporary Decline, and Recurrence

Healing rarely follows a perfectly rising line. Stress, grief, illness, pain, insomnia, psychiatric symptoms, reduced treatment engagement, relationship conflict, or cue exposure may temporarily lower reserve. The patient may need a return to greater structure, medication review, reduced responsibility, or more intensive treatment.

A temporary decline does not erase prior learning, relationships, insight, or capacity. Recurrence may indicate that the prior protection plan was insufficient for the conditions that developed and warrants serious reassessment.

Progress can remain real even when the patient temporarily needs more help.

Selected supporting evidence: [63–64,91].

Measurement and Future Research

There is currently no clinical “glucometer” for Homeostatic Reserve or the Healing Trajectory. The framework does not claim that one score can measure the patient’s position, validate a threshold, or predict recurrence.

Potential research domains include sleep and circadian stability, autonomic regulation, executive function, hedonic tone, stress reactivity, emotional regulation, psychiatric stability, social connection, treatment participation, recovery-capital use, functional behavior, and value-congruent action. These are candidate domains for study rather than elements of a provisional composite score. Repeated measurement across time may eventually help determine which combinations best represent meaningful changes in reserve and trajectory.

The framework should therefore be treated as a hypothesis-generating conceptual model until its domains, relationships, thresholds, trajectories, and clinical applications are formally operationalized and studied.

Selected supporting evidence: [3,58,61–62].

The Reserve–Threshold–Trajectory Architecture

In summary, Reserve names available capacity, Threshold names functional position, and Trajectory names change over time.

Selected supporting evidence: [2,10,52,60].

Chapter 6 Closing Perspective

Healing follows a trajectory, not a stopwatch.

The next chapter translates the Healing Trajectory into multidisciplinary, stage-matched treatment: what the team provides, how therapeutic methods should change, and when deeper work becomes more usable.

Chapter Summary

The Homeostatic Reserve Healing Trajectory adds time to the model. Recovery is nonlinear, multidomain, and heterogeneous: acute stabilization may occur before executive function, reward responsiveness, relationships, identity, and meaning have recovered sufficiently for independent living. Treatment should therefore change as the patient's capacity changes.

Key Clinical Takeaways

- The four phases are heuristic guideposts rather than biological deadlines.
- Different systems heal at different rates, and external scaffolding may remain necessary after abstinence is established.
- The clinical approach should change as capacity changes: concrete and protective early, increasingly skills based and direct during rebuilding, and deeper when regulation is sufficiently durable.
- Recurrence warrants serious reassessment but does not prove that one specific element of the prior plan failed.

Chapter 7 — Effective Treatment: Multidisciplinary, Stage-Matched Care

How Coordinated Treatment Scaffolds Recovery While Capacity Is Rebuilt

Addictive illness affects physiology, motivation, learning, stress, cognition, relationships, judgment, and the patient's ability to use help. Effective treatment must therefore be broader than withdrawal management, medication alone, individual psychotherapy alone, or simple removal from substance access. It requires a coordinated plan that addresses the illness as it is expressed in the whole person.

The strongest treatment programs do not merely assemble many services. They organize those services around a shared clinical formulation. Medicine, nursing, psychotherapy, addiction counseling, family work, group treatment, peer support, case management, and recovery planning should reinforce one another rather than operate as disconnected interventions.

> *Effective treatment is not one profession doing everything. It is a coordinated team doing the right things, in the right sequence, at the level of intensity the patient can currently use.*

Selected supporting evidence: [32,36,63–66,69,92,94].

Why Addictive Illness Requires a Multidisciplinary Response

A person may enter treatment with withdrawal, sleep deprivation, pain, malnutrition, trauma-related arousal, depression, mania, anxiety, cognitive impairment, family conflict, occupational consequences, unstable housing, and a deeply conditioned pattern of relief seeking. No single discipline is positioned to evaluate and treat all of these domains well.

A physician may stabilize withdrawal and prescribe evidence-based medication, but medication does not by itself teach the patient how to identify cues, disclose risk, repair relationships, tolerate shame, or build a recovery life. A therapist may help the patient understand trauma, grief, and emotional patterns, but psychotherapy is less effective when intoxication, withdrawal, severe insomnia, uncontrolled pain, or psychiatric instability repeatedly overwhelms attention and regulation. A counselor may translate illness understanding into daily recovery behavior, but counseling cannot substitute for medical treatment when withdrawal or co-occurring illness creates biological danger. Peer support can make recovery believable, but peers should not be asked to perform diagnosis, medication management, emergency care, or psychotherapy.

The purpose of the team is not to divide the patient into separate problems. It is to create one coordinated treatment environment in which each discipline addresses the part of the illness it is trained to treat while contributing to a shared recovery plan.

> *The patient experiences one illness across many domains. The team must provide one coordinated response across many disciplines.*

Selected supporting evidence: [32,64–66,92,94].

The First Requirement: Interrupt the Pattern Long Enough for Treatment to Work

Psychotherapy, counseling, family work, and recovery education require some minimum capacity for attention, memory, emotional tolerance, and participation. When repeated intoxication, withdrawal, cue exposure, sleep disruption, or immediate access continually resets the patient into crisis, treatment cannot accumulate.

The offending substance or pattern of use must therefore be interrupted long enough for the patient to become medically safer and sufficiently regulated to participate. For some substances, this requires medically managed withdrawal. For others, it requires medication treatment, access restriction, monitoring, a structured living environment, or a higher level of care. Interruption is not the whole treatment, but it creates the protected interval in which treatment can begin to have a cumulative effect.

The goal is not simply to produce days without use. The protected time should be used to restore sleep, stabilize medical and psychiatric symptoms, begin medication when indicated, establish predictable routines, reduce exposure to high-risk cues, and introduce the patient to the relationships and practices that will support continuing recovery.

> *Removing the substance can stop the immediate cycle. Effective treatment uses the interruption to build the capacity that makes continued recovery possible.*

Selected supporting evidence: [32,36,63–64,92,94].

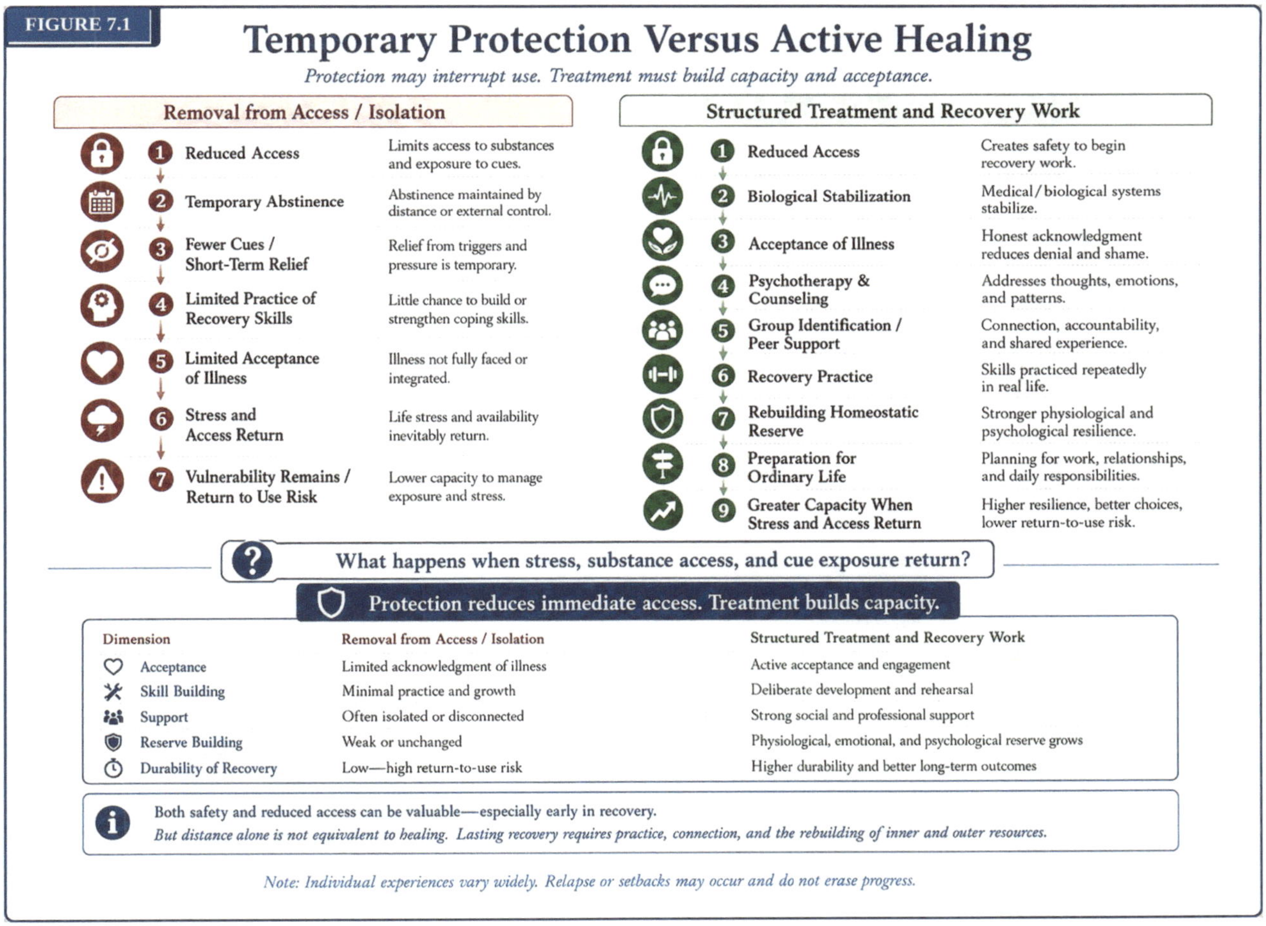

Figure 7.1. Temporary Protection Versus Active Healing. Temporary removal from substance access and cues may interrupt use, while structured treatment can use protected time to build acceptance, regulation, recovery skills, relationships, and preparation for the return of stress, availability, and cue exposure. This figure is a conceptual educational representation, not a validated treatment algorithm or measurement instrument. Homeostatic Reserve represents integrated regulatory capacity, not a literal dopamine or neurotransmitter supply. Supporting evidence for component mechanisms: [32,63,94].

Two Common Starting Sequences—and No Universal Order

Many patients enter treatment through one of two broad clinical sequences. These sequences are useful for planning, but they are not rigid categories and should not be treated as universal rules.

When addictive illness is the dominant destabilizing force

In some patients, the substance pattern is driving most of the acute instability. Withdrawal, intoxication, cue-driven behavior, sleep loss, secrecy, and repeated relief seeking are amplifying anxiety, depression, irritability, cognitive impairment, and family conflict. The initial treatment emphasis should be on interrupting use, managing withdrawal, restoring sleep, reducing access, beginning medication when indicated, and establishing enough structure for the patient to participate.

Early psychotherapy in this sequence is often supportive, motivational, educational, and skills focused. The patient may first need help understanding what is happening, tolerating the treatment environment, accepting assistance, identifying immediate risk, and learning basic cognitive and behavioral strategies. As capacity improves, therapy can become more exploratory and more directly focused on illness recognition, consequences, relational patterns, grief, trauma, and repair.

When psychiatric or trauma-related flooding is the dominant destabilizing force

Other patients arrive so flooded by panic, trauma activation, severe depression, mania, psychosis, dissociation, suicidality, or another mental health condition that they cannot meaningfully engage in addiction treatment until the acute psychiatric state is stabilized. In these situations, psychiatric safety and symptom stabilization may be the immediate priority.

This does not mean the addictive illness should be ignored while mental health treatment proceeds. Continuing substance exposure may worsen the psychiatric syndrome, obscure diagnosis, impair medication response, and repeatedly destabilize the patient. The treatment plan should therefore interrupt the substance pattern while simultaneously addressing the condition that is preventing participation.

The central principle is integrated care rather than a contest over which diagnosis is primary. The first priority is the condition that is most threatening to safety or most responsible for making treatment inaccessible, while both disorders remain visible in the same formulation.

> *There is no universal addiction-first or trauma-first sequence. The sequence should begin with what must be stabilized for the patient to become safe and able to participate—while the substance pattern is interrupted and both conditions remain in treatment.*

Selected supporting evidence: [71–72,92,94].

Treatment as Coordinated Scaffolding

Within the Homeostatic Reserve Model, treatment can provide temporary external scaffolding while internal capacity is insufficient. The treatment environment may organize sleep, meals, medication, monitoring, transportation, appointments, access restriction, emotional containment, and recovery practice. The team may recognize danger before the patient can recognize it, hold hope when the patient cannot feel it, and maintain structure when the patient cannot yet create it independently.

This scaffolding should not be confused with passivity or permanent dependence. Its purpose is to protect the patient long enough for functions to be practiced and gradually internalized. The patient begins by borrowing structure, interpretation, accountability, and regulation from the environment. Over time, they learn to recognize warning signs, protect sleep, use medication responsibly, ask for help earlier, tolerate emotion, and make recovery-supportive decisions with less external prompting.

Treatment initially supplies functions the depleted patient cannot yet perform reliably. Recovery allows the patient to gradually reclaim those functions.

Selected supporting evidence: [32,36,63,69,94]. The treatment-scaffolding relationship is an original clinical proposition within the Homeostatic Reserve Model.

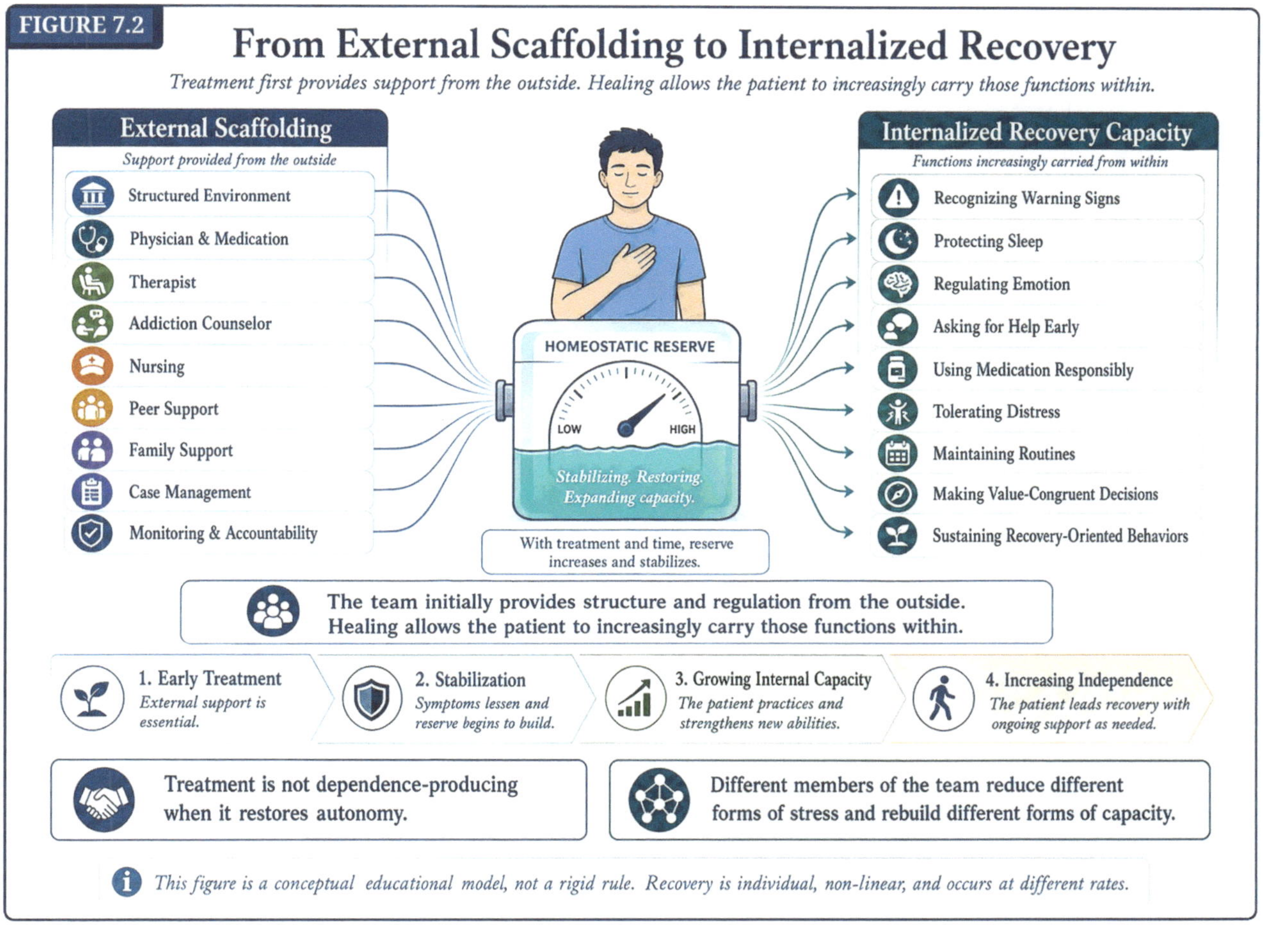

Figure 7.2. From External Scaffolding to Internalized Recovery. Within the model, the treatment team may initially provide structure, regulation, monitoring, interpretation, accountability, and support from the outside. Healing may allow the patient to increasingly recognize risk, regulate emotion, use support, protect recovery, and carry these functions within. This figure is a conceptual educational representation, not a validated measurement of internalization. Homeostatic Reserve represents integrated regulatory capacity, not a literal dopamine or neurotransmitter supply. Supporting evidence for component mechanisms: [36,63,69].

Trust, Rapport, and Range: The Relational Scaffold

In early treatment, one of the treatment team's most important tasks is to build trust with the patient and, when clinically appropriate and authorized, with the family or other key supports. Trust is not a sentimental extra added after "real" treatment. It is part of the treatment environment that allows the patient to tolerate evaluation, remain engaged, accept structure, disclose risk, and eventually examine illness-related distortions without experiencing every intervention as attack.

Trust usually develops gradually. In the first days or weeks, the team builds it through reliability, consistency, accurate information, respectful limit-setting, confidentiality boundaries, attention to immediate suffering, and follow-through on what has been promised. Family trust is built in a similar way: by explaining the treatment frame, clarifying what can and cannot be shared, acknowledging fear and exhaustion, and helping loved ones understand how support, boundaries, and safety planning can work together.

A safe treatment environment does not mean that distorted perceptions, minimization, rationalization, dishonesty, or avoidance are never challenged. It means that challenge is delivered at the right time, with the right level of directness, by a professional who has enough rapport to make the intervention usable. When the patient's reserve is low, the team may need to begin with stabilization, motivational engagement, concrete feedback, and repeated orientation. As capacity and trust improve, the same team may be able to ask more probing questions, name contradictions more directly, and help the patient accept the diagnosis and its consequences.

This combination of rapport and range is a marker of professional maturity. Rapport allows the clinician to be trusted enough to influence the patient. Range allows the clinician to shift stance across patients, families, cultures, stages of illness, and stages of healing. Some patients require gentle motivational engagement before direct confrontation is useful. Others need firm, immediate structure because risk is high. Diverse populations may require different language, cultural humility, attention to prior experiences with healthcare systems, and awareness of how authority, shame, stigma, family roles, spirituality, gender, race, occupation, or trauma history affect whether help feels safe.

> *Trust does not replace clinical truth. It creates the relational safety and credibility needed for truth to become usable.*

Selected supporting evidence: [69,71,88,92,94,97–99].

The Multidisciplinary Treatment Team

Not every patient requires every professional at every stage, but severe addictive illness commonly requires expertise from several disciplines. The essential feature is not the number of team members. It is whether the necessary functions are present, coordinated, and responsive to the patient's changing needs.

Addiction medicine and psychiatric care

Physicians and advanced practice clinicians evaluate intoxication and withdrawal risk, medical illness, pain, sleep, cognition, medication interactions, psychiatric symptoms, and the possibility of substance-induced syndromes. They initiate and monitor evidence-based medication when indicated, treat co-occurring illness, and help distinguish symptoms that improve with abstinence from conditions requiring continuing treatment.

Nursing and day-to-day clinical observation

Nurses provide monitoring, medication administration, patient education, consistency, early recognition of change, and repeated contact across the day. Because they often observe sleep, appetite, autonomic symptoms, medication response, interpersonal behavior, and fluctuations in distress, nursing observations can reveal patterns that are not visible in a scheduled interview.

Individual psychotherapy

Individual therapy provides a confidential setting to examine the patient's particular history, emotions, beliefs, defenses, relationships, trauma, grief, and patterns of relief seeking. Early work may emphasize alliance, trust, stabilization, motivational enhancement, psychoeducation, and concrete coping. Later work may become more interpretive, more direct, and more focused on acceptance, identity, responsibility, repair, and grief or trauma at a depth the patient can safely tolerate.

Addiction counseling and recovery skill development

Addiction counselors help translate the illness formulation into daily behavior. They teach cue recognition, craving management, cognitive and behavioral skills, recovery routines, relapse-prevention planning, use of support, and practical responses to high-risk situations. They also help the patient connect consequences that were previously experienced as separate events into one understandable illness pattern.

Group therapy and the therapeutic community

Group treatment allows patients to learn from one another, recognize shared patterns, receive feedback, practice honesty, experience accountability, and observe recovery in other people. A well-led group can reduce shame without minimizing responsibility. It can also reveal how the patient responds to frustration, difference, limits, vulnerability, and interpersonal feedback.

Group placement and intensity should be matched to cognitive capacity, psychiatric stability, safety, and readiness. Group therapy is not automatically appropriate in every acute state, and poorly timed or poorly led confrontation can increase defensiveness rather than insight.

Family therapy and family education

Addictive illness reorganizes family life. Loved ones may become frightened, controlling, avoidant, overfunctioning, secretive, or exhausted. Family treatment can clarify the illness, improve communication, establish boundaries, reduce behaviors that unintentionally maintain risk, and create a safer plan for continuing recovery. It also helps the team build trust with family members so that support and accountability are less likely to be experienced as punishment, rescue, or confusion.

Family involvement must remain individualized. The patient should help define whom they consider family. The team must also consider confidentiality, withdrawal status, co-occurring illness, violence, coercion, estrangement, and whether contact with particular relatives is stabilizing or harmful. Family therapy is a treatment modality—not a requirement that every relationship be restored.

Peer support and recovery mentorship

Peers and recovery coaches contribute identification, practical experience, hope, community connection, and visible evidence that a meaningful recovery life is possible. They may help patients learn how to use mutual-support groups, navigate early recovery, build routines, and tolerate the unfamiliarity of living without the substance.

Peer support complements professional treatment but does not replace medical care, psychotherapy, emergency response, or formal risk assessment. Clear role boundaries protect both the patient and the peer relationship.

Case management and environmental stabilization

Housing, transportation, finances, legal obligations, access to medication, employment, childcare, and continuity of care can consume enough reserve to undermine otherwise effective treatment. Case managers help reduce these practical barriers and coordinate transitions so that gains made in structure are not immediately overwhelmed by an unstable environment.

Dietitians, occupational therapists, physical therapists, exercise professionals, chaplains, vocational specialists, and other clinicians may also contribute when nutrition, physical functioning, pain, spirituality, work, or another domain is clinically important.

> *The team does more than reduce symptoms. It helps make recovery medically safer, psychologically understandable, behaviorally practicable, relationally supported, and increasingly livable.*

Selected supporting evidence: [36,65–66,90,92,94,97].

Different Modalities Perform Different Functions

Effective treatment is not defined by offering every modality to every patient. It is defined by selecting interventions that address the patient's current risks and needs, delivering them with adequate intensity, and changing the plan as the patient's capacity and circumstances change.

- Medication may reduce withdrawal, craving, physiologic instability, psychiatric symptoms, pain, or sleep disruption and thereby reduce pressures that repeatedly pull reserve downward.
- Motivational approaches can strengthen engagement and help the patient examine ambivalence without humiliation or coercive confrontation.
- Cognitive and behavioral therapies can help the patient identify thoughts, cues, routines, and consequences while practicing alternative responses.
- Contingency-based and behavioral interventions can reinforce recovery-supportive actions when the delayed benefits of recovery are not yet strongly felt.
- Individual therapy can address the patient's unique history, emotional burden, defenses, identity, and relationships.
- Group therapy can provide identification, feedback, belonging, accountability, and repeated interpersonal practice.
- Family therapy can alter the relational environment in which illness and recovery occur.
- Peer and mutual support can extend recovery beyond professional treatment and provide continuing community.
- Case management can make treatment usable by reducing environmental barriers and coordinating care.

A treatment plan is strongest when the team can explain what each intervention is intended to accomplish, how progress will be recognized, and what change in the patient's condition would require the plan to be intensified, modified, or simplified.

Selected supporting evidence: [36,63,65–69,92,94,97].

Stage-Matched Treatment Across the Healing Trajectory

The same patient may need very different treatment during the first week, the eighth week, and the sixth month. This difference should not be interpreted as inconsistency. It reflects the fact that the patient's available capacity, risks, insight, trust in the team, and ability to use treatment are changing.

The phases below are heuristic and overlapping. They do not establish fixed timelines or require every patient to progress in the same order.

Stage-Matched Multidisciplinary Treatment Across the Healing Trajectory

Treatment emphasis changes as safety, regulation, and functional capacity become more reliable.

ILLUSTRATIVE TREATMENT PHASES	PHASE 1 Acute stabilization Days to early weeks	PHASE 2 Early rebuilding Several weeks	PHASE 3 Consolidation Weeks to months	PHASE 4 Integration Months and beyond
	MORE EXTERNAL SUPPORT →			→ MORE INTERNALIZED CAPACITY
Homeostatic Reserve	Low / highly supported	Beginning to rebuild	More durable	Greater internal capacity
Primary clinical focus	Safety and stabilization	Restore basic regulation	Illness work and skill integration	Meaning, repair, and long-term living
Team emphasis	Medical and nursing stabilization; predictable structure	Counseling, groups, medication optimization, family education	More direct therapy, relapse analysis, relationship work	Individualized trauma/grief work, family repair, community and vocation
Therapeutic stance	Concrete, calm, repetitive, nonshaming	Collaborative, skills focused, increasingly direct	Direct, curious, accountable, emotionally tolerable	Deeper and exploratory, matched to stability and preference

Good treatment meets the patient where capacity is, supplies what is temporarily missing, and changes as the patient becomes able to carry more of recovery internally.

Figure 7.3. Stage-Matched Multidisciplinary Treatment Across the Healing Trajectory. The figure presents illustrative, overlapping treatment phases rather than fixed timelines or a validated treatment algorithm. Clinical sequencing should remain individualized, guideline-concordant, and responsive to safety, co-occurring conditions, patient preference, and demonstrated function. Supporting evidence for component mechanisms: [32,63,65–66,69,71–72,92,94,97].

Acute stabilization: make treatment possible

During the first days or weeks, the patient may be sleep deprived, frightened, cognitively slowed, emotionally labile, medically unstable, or preoccupied with immediate relief. The treatment should be concrete and repetitive. The patient may need information presented more than once. Expectations should be clear, routines predictable, trust actively built, and feedback focused on immediate safety and participation.

This is rarely the ideal moment for prolonged interpretive therapy, aggressive confrontation, or detailed exploration of every traumatic experience. The patient is not being protected from truth. The truth is being delivered in a form and sequence the patient can currently use.

Early rebuilding: teach skills before demanding mastery

As sleep, withdrawal, and acute psychiatric symptoms improve, the patient can begin learning more complex skills. Cognitive and behavioral strategies, motivational work, group participation, cue recognition, emotional labeling, family education, and structured recovery practice become more useful.

The patient may still rely heavily on the team to identify patterns and organize action. Success at this stage should be measured partly by willingness to participate, disclose, practice, and accept help—not only by the sophistication of insight.

Consolidation: use improved capacity for more direct illness work

By the eighth or twelfth week, some patients—but not all—have accumulated enough sleep, abstinence, medication response, group experience, and cognitive-behavioral practice to tolerate more probing questions and more direct feedback. They may be increasingly able to examine minimization, connect consequences, recognize the illness across time, understand the effects on others, and consider changes that previously felt unbearable.

Directness should remain collaborative rather than punitive. The purpose is not to defeat the patient in an argument. It is to help the patient see a pattern clearly enough to protect themselves from it.

Integration: approach grief, trauma, and identity at the right depth

As regulation becomes more durable, the patient may be able to engage more fully with grief, trauma, shame, chronic pain, family history, identity, intimacy, or meaning. These issues may have preceded the addiction, resulted from it, or both. Addressing them can reduce suffering and strengthen long-term recovery.

Deeper work should not be postponed by a rigid rule requiring a predetermined period of abstinence, nor should it be initiated simply because a calendar date has arrived. The depth and pacing should be matched to safety, psychiatric stability, emotional tolerance, coping capacity, patient preference, and the support available during and after the work. Integrated trauma-focused treatment may be appropriate when those conditions are present.

> *The treatment should not be less honest early in recovery. It should be more carefully timed, more concrete, and better matched to the patient's capacity to use what is being offered.*

Selected supporting evidence: [63,69,71–72,92,94].

Direct Questioning, Feedback, and Therapeutic Timing

Patients with severe addictive illness often need help seeing patterns they cannot yet organize independently. Effective treatment should not avoid difficult information, but the manner, timing, and relational foundation of feedback strongly influence whether it becomes usable.

Early in treatment, questions may need to be concrete: What happened? What did you use? When did sleep change? What was the consequence? Who knew? What help was available? Later, the team can ask more integrative questions: What did you believe at the time? What pattern connects these events? How did the illness change what felt important? What would accepting the diagnosis require you to do differently?

Collaborative feedback identifies discrepancy without attacking identity. It combines compassion with accountability and distinguishes explanation from excuse. Rapport makes the feedback more likely to be heard; range allows the professional to adjust directness, pacing, and modality for the patient's culture, history, current reserve, family context, and stage of healing. The patient can be treated as a good person with a powerful illness while still being expected to tell the truth, protect others, repair harm where possible, and participate in the work required for recovery.

> *The goal of direct feedback is not to break the patient down. It is to help the patient build enough clarity to stop being repeatedly defeated by the same illness pattern.*

Selected supporting evidence: [69,73–74,92].

Team Coherence: One Formulation, Many Disciplines

A multidisciplinary program can still fail if the team communicates poorly, sends contradictory messages, or treats each problem in isolation. Effective teams share a working formulation, define responsibilities, communicate clinically important changes, and agree on the major treatment priorities.

Rapport and range

The clinical capacity to build enough trust and credibility for difficult interventions to be usable while also shifting stance, language, modality, directness, and pacing across diverse patients, families, cultures, stages of illness, and stages of healing.

Therapeutic alliance

The collaborative relationship that supports engagement, safety, disclosure, motivation, and shared work toward recovery goals. Within this book, alliance is not a substitute for accountability; it is part of the clinical environment that makes accountability more usable.

Team coherence does not require every clinician to use the same modality. It requires that different modalities move in the same direction. The physician's medication plan, the therapist's work, the counselor's recovery assignments, the family plan, the peer-support strategy, and the discharge plan should not undermine one another.

The patient and family, when involved with consent and appropriate boundaries, should also understand the plan. Whenever possible, the team should explain what is being treated, why each service is being recommended, what progress would look like, what information can and cannot be shared, and what signs would indicate the need for more support.

> *The patient should not have to assemble the treatment plan from separate conversations. The team should present one understandable path through care.*

Selected supporting evidence: [32,92,94].

Function-Based Progression Through Care

The amount of time spent in treatment matters, but time alone does not establish readiness for less structure. A patient may appear stable because the environment is carrying substantial regulatory load. Progression should therefore consider what the patient can do reliably as scaffolding is reduced.

Relevant evidence may include stable sleep, medical and psychiatric regulation, medication adherence, improving cognition, honest disclosure, use of support, ability to tolerate frustration, recovery behavior outside direct supervision, response to cue exposure, family observations, and performance during increasing responsibility. Transitions should follow current ASAM standards and individualized clinical judgment rather than a fixed program calendar.

A temporary return to greater structure should not be interpreted as failure. It may be the treatment response required when stress rises, reserve falls, psychiatric symptoms intensify, or the patient encounters demands they cannot yet manage safely.

> *The question is not only whether the patient can succeed inside structure. It is whether enough of that success has become durable when structure is gradually reduced.*

Selected supporting evidence: [32,63–64,94].

What Effective Treatment Is Not

- It is not withdrawal management presented as complete treatment.
- It is not simple isolation from substances without active skill building and preparation for ordinary life.
- It is not one profession attempting to perform every clinical function.
- It is not the same sequence, modality, or length of care for every patient.
- It is not indefinite postponement of trauma, grief, or psychiatric treatment until an arbitrary abstinence milestone.

- It is not premature deep exploration that overwhelms the patient's current capacity for safety and regulation.
- It is not confrontation designed to humiliate, overpower, or force verbal agreement.
- It is not peer support used as a substitute for medical or psychotherapeutic care.
- It is not compassion without accountability or accountability without compassion.

Effective treatment is coordinated, evidence based, person centered, sufficiently intensive, and responsive to change. It protects the patient while capacity is low, uses the protected time to build capacity, and progressively transfers responsibility back to the patient as that capacity becomes more reliable.

Selected supporting evidence: [32,63–66,69,71–72,92,94].

Integrating Effective Treatment With the Reserve–Threshold–Trajectory Architecture

The Homeostatic Reserve Model offers a practical way to understand why the same modality may be useful at one point and ineffective or destabilizing at another. Treatment should be matched not only to diagnosis, but also to the patient's current functional capacity, position relative to the conceptual threshold, and movement along the healing trajectory.

Below the threshold, the patient may need greater external structure, simpler interventions, more repetition, reduced access, medication, and immediate support. Near the threshold, the patient may begin practicing more independent regulation while still requiring rapid access to the team. Above the threshold, the patient may be better able to tolerate direct feedback, use insight, engage natural reward, repair relationships, and sustain value-congruent action—but vulnerability has not disappeared.

The model does not determine a level of care or prescribe a specific treatment sequence. It provides a language for asking whether the patient currently has enough capacity to use what is being offered and what forms of scaffolding are still necessary.

> *Good treatment meets the patient where their capacity is, supplies what is temporarily missing, and changes as the patient becomes able to carry more of recovery within themselves.*

Selected supporting evidence for component mechanisms: [32,36,63,69,92,94]. The integrated Reserve–Threshold–Trajectory treatment relationship remains an original proposition of the Homeostatic Reserve Model.

Chapter 7 Closing Perspective

Effective treatment interrupts the substance pattern, stabilizes what is most dangerous, builds trust with the patient and family, and surrounds the patient with enough medical, psychological, relational, and environmental support for healing to accumulate. It recognizes that patients do not have the same capacity during the first week that they may have during the eighth or twelfth week. It therefore changes its methods as the patient changes.

Early treatment may be more protective, concrete, repetitive, and externally structured. Later treatment may become more direct, more exploratory, and more focused on grief, trauma, responsibility, repair, identity, and meaning. Neither phase is more legitimate. Each is appropriate to a different clinical state.

> *The best treatment does not merely ask the patient to make better choices. It helps restore the capacity required to make those choices—and then teaches the patient how to protect that capacity over time.*

Chapter Summary

- Effective treatment is multidisciplinary because addictive illness affects biological, psychiatric, cognitive, motivational, relational, and environmental functioning.

- The substance pattern must be interrupted long enough for treatment to accumulate, but interruption alone is not complete treatment.
- There is no universal addiction-first or trauma-first sequence. The initial priority is the condition most threatening to safety or treatment participation while both disorders remain integrated in the plan.
- Treatment provides external scaffolding when reserve is low and progressively transfers regulatory functions back to the patient as capacity improves.
- Medicine, nursing, psychotherapy, counseling, groups, family therapy, peer support, and case management contribute different functions and require coordination.
- The therapeutic approach should change across the Healing Trajectory: concrete and protective early, increasingly direct and skills based during rebuilding, and deeper and more exploratory as regulation becomes durable.
- Building trust with the patient and family is an early treatment priority because trust helps create the safe environment in which disclosure, feedback, accountability, and deeper therapeutic work become usable.
- Rapport and range allow professionals to challenge distorted perceptions at the right time and to adjust modality, language, directness, and pacing across diverse populations and stages of illness and healing.
- Progression through care should follow demonstrated function, evolving need, current standards, and clinical judgment—not time alone.

Key Clinical Takeaways

- Ask not only what diagnosis is present, but what the patient can currently use.
- Stabilize whatever is preventing safety and participation while interrupting the substance pattern.
- Do not confuse early cognitive or emotional limitation with unwillingness alone.
- Build trust deliberately with the patient and family while maintaining confidentiality, safety, and clear clinical boundaries.
- Do not confuse a safe environment with avoidance of difficult truth; challenge distortions when rapport, capacity, and timing make the intervention usable.
- Use direct feedback collaboratively and increase depth, probing, and challenge as trust and capacity make the intervention more usable.
- Treat trauma and grief when clinically appropriate; neither postpone them by rigid rule nor pursue them at a depth the patient cannot safely sustain.
- Coordinate the team so that medication, therapy, counseling, family work, peer support, and discharge planning reinforce one understandable treatment path.
- Treatment makes the fight more fair by reducing destabilizing pressures, providing temporary scaffolding, and rebuilding the capacity for value-congruent action.

The next chapter turns from the architecture of treatment to the specific domains through which Homeostatic Reserve is progressively rebuilt.

Chapter 8 — Rebuilding Homeostatic Reserve

How Treatment Restores Capacity for Regulation, Choice, and Meaningful Living

Abstinence may interrupt one of the largest ongoing sources of depletion and is central to many recovery pathways. Within the Homeostatic Reserve Model, durable recovery is conceptualized as multidomain rebuilding through biological stabilization, restorative sleep, indicated medication, emotional regulation, structured behavior, supportive relationships, meaningful activity, natural reward, and time. The relative contribution of each domain varies by patient.

Stopping depletion is not the same as rebuilding capacity.

Supporting evidence for component mechanisms: [57–58,63,94]. These sources support component mechanisms; the model's integrated relationship remains an original conceptual proposition.

Rebuilding Is Multidomain

The model treats recovery capacity as the integrated result of biological regulation, sleep, psychiatric stability, cognition, emotion, physical health, relationships, environmental safety, recovery skills, meaning, and repeated value-congruent behavior. No single domain is sufficient, and the construct has not been validated as a composite measure.

Weakness in one domain increases strain on others. Poor sleep worsens anxiety, pain, attention, irritability, craving, and conflict. Conflict then worsens sleep. Untreated pain may impair movement, mood, work, relationships, and hope.

Because the domains interact, one unresolved drain can amplify several others.

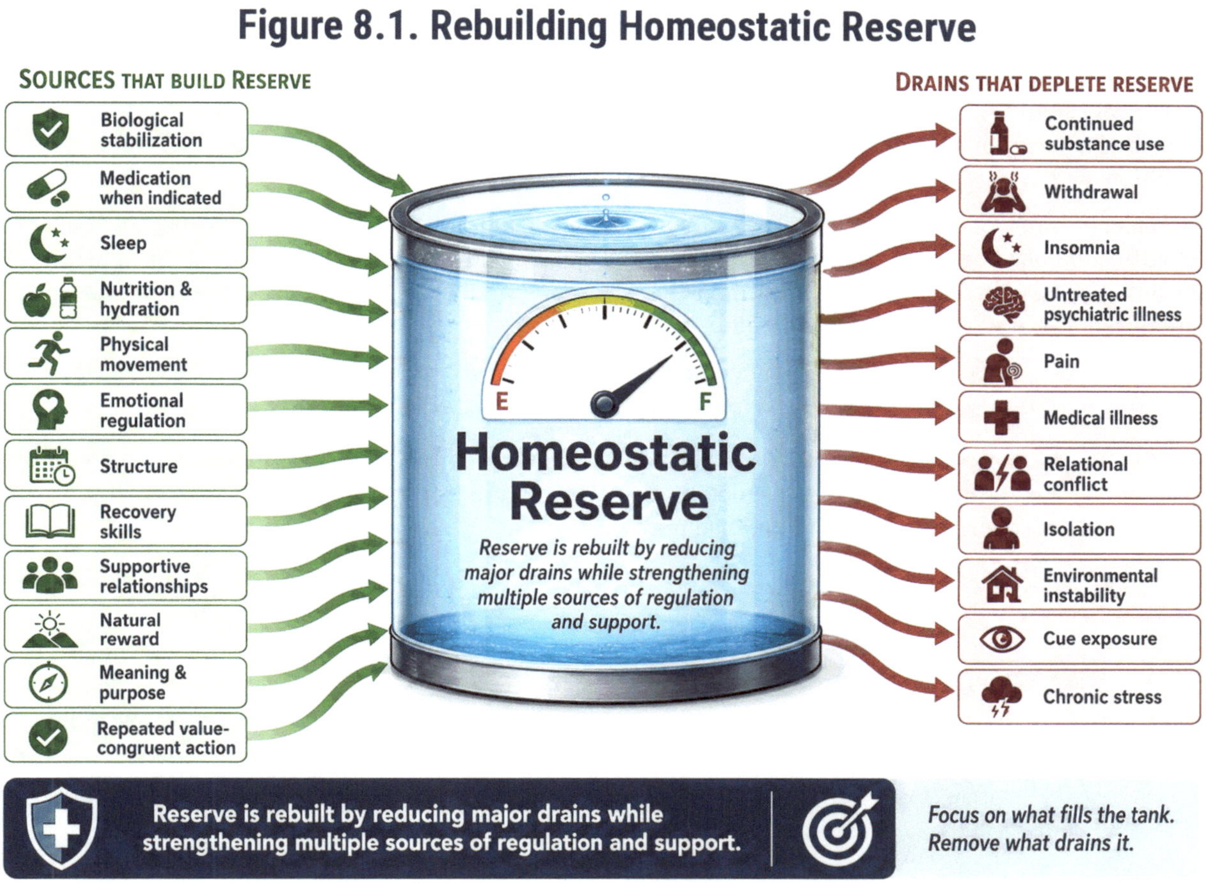

Figure 8.1. Rebuilding Homeostatic Reserve. Within the model, reserve may rebuild as major drains are reduced and biological stability, sleep, health, emotional regulation, structure, recovery skills, supportive relationships, natural reward, meaning, and value-congruent action strengthen. This figure is a conceptual educational representation, not a validated measurement instrument, treatment sequence, or universal recovery pathway. Homeostatic Reserve represents integrated regulatory capacity, not a literal dopamine or neurotransmitter supply. Supporting evidence for component mechanisms: [57–58,60,63].

Supporting evidence for component mechanisms: [57–58,60,63]. These sources support component mechanisms; the model's integrated relationship remains an original conceptual proposition.

The First Task Is to Stop Major Leaks

Early rebuilding often requires identifying and reducing the largest sources of ongoing depletion. These may include continued exposure, withdrawal, severe insomnia, untreated depression or anxiety, mania or psychosis, uncontrolled pain, nutritional deficits, medical illness, relational chaos, legal crisis, unsafe housing, and repeated cue exposure. Priorities should be individualized according to safety and clinical need.

Early treatment therefore often feels practical rather than inspirational. It may begin with safety, sleep, nutrition, medication, reduced access, urgent medical care, and predictable structure.

> *Rebuilding is difficult while the largest sources of depletion remain active.*

Selected supporting evidence: [34,36,92,94].

Biological Stabilization

Biological stabilization provides the foundation for later treatment. The patient may need support for withdrawal, autonomic instability, sleep disruption, appetite, nutrition, pain, mood symptoms, anxiety, cognition, and medical illness.

For patients at risk of clinically significant withdrawal, medication-assisted withdrawal management during the detoxification phase may be necessary to reduce suffering, prevent complications, and create sufficient physiological stability for meaningful participation. The appropriate level of care depends on the substance, anticipated withdrawal severity, comorbidity, history, and current findings.

> *Detoxification addresses the acute physiological consequences of stopping a substance. Comprehensive treatment addresses the illness that made continued use difficult to stop.*

A patient who is sleep-deprived, withdrawing, panicked, depressed, psychotic, or cognitively impaired may be less able to retain information, regulate emotion, participate in group, understand consequences, or use coping skills. Capacity should be assessed rather than presumed absent.

Selected supporting evidence: [34–36,92].

Medication and Structure as Scaffolding

When indicated, medication may reduce specific pressures such as withdrawal, craving, mood instability, anxiety, psychosis, insomnia, pain, or attentional symptoms. Medication does not replace recovery work, and effects vary by diagnosis, medication, adherence, patient, and setting. It may make particular forms of recovery work more accessible.

> *Within the Homeostatic Reserve Model, structure can scaffold behavior from the outside; indicated medication can scaffold regulation from the inside.*

The purpose of scaffolding is not dependence on treatment. It is restoration of the capacity needed for increasing independence.

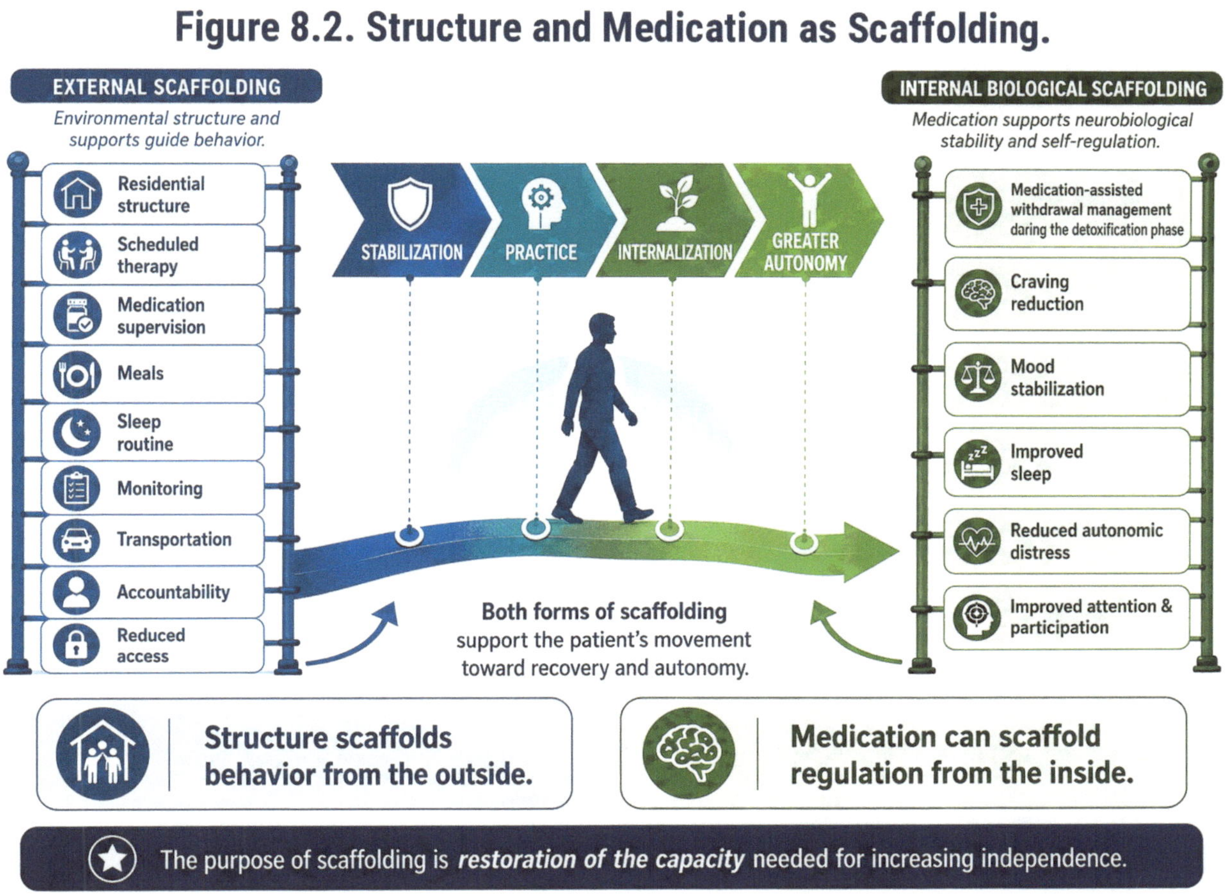

Figure 8.2. Structure and Medication as Scaffolding. Within the model, structure may scaffold behavior from the outside, while indicated medication may scaffold regulation from the inside. Stabilization can create opportunities for practice, internalization, and increasing autonomy. This figure is a conceptual educational representation, not a validated treatment algorithm or measure of dependence or readiness. Homeostatic Reserve represents integrated regulatory capacity, not a literal dopamine or neurotransmitter supply. Supporting evidence for component mechanisms: [36–37,39,63].

Supporting evidence for component mechanisms: [36–37,39–41]. These sources support component mechanisms; the model's integrated relationship remains an original conceptual proposition.

Sleep, Nutrition, Movement, and Physical Restoration

Sleep is an important reserve-supporting domain. Poor sleep may worsen mood, anxiety, pain, memory, impulse control, craving, emotional reactivity, and interpretation of stress, although the magnitude and direction of these relationships vary.

> *Sleep does not solve every problem, but without adequate sleep many problems become harder to solve.*

Some patients enter treatment with nutritional deficits, dehydration, or untreated medical conditions. Regular meals, hydration, correction of identified deficiencies, and medical treatment can reduce avoidable biological demand. Appropriately prescribed movement may support sleep, mood, routine, confidence, physical health, natural reward, and social connection; direct effects on substance-use outcomes are heterogeneous.

Movement can help the patient experience the body as a source of regulation rather than only a source of craving, pain, or distress.

Selected supporting evidence: [20,55–56,94].

Structure Is Borrowed Reserve

Early in recovery, some patients may not yet be able to organize life reliably. A structured environment can temporarily provide predictable sleep and wake times, medication adherence, meals, therapy, group attendance, transportation, accountability, and reduced exposure.

Within the Homeostatic Reserve Model, structure may function as borrowed reserve.

Improvement within structure does not automatically establish readiness to function with less support because the environment may be carrying substantial regulatory load. Transitions should follow current authoritative level-of-care criteria and individualized clinical judgment, based on demonstrated function and evolving need rather than impatience or an arbitrary duration.

Supporting evidence for component mechanisms: [32,63,94]. These sources support component mechanisms; the model's integrated relationship remains an original conceptual proposition.

Repetition Builds Capacity

Recovery skills become reliable through repetition. The patient may need repeated practice recognizing craving, identifying emotion, tolerating distress, contacting support, challenging distorted thinking, setting boundaries, protecting sleep, using medication responsibly, and leaving high-risk situations.

Understanding a skill once is not the same as using it under stress.

Knowledge becomes capacity only through repeated application.

Selected supporting evidence: [65,69,91].

Relationships, Natural Reward, Meaning, and Self-Respect

Safe relationships may provide emotional containment, feedback, encouragement, accountability, belonging, practical help, and protection against isolation. Natural reward may return gradually and unevenly. A patient may intellectually understand that relationships, exercise, work, music, nature, creativity, spirituality, or service are valuable before being able to feel their value fully.

Behavioral recovery may precede the return of felt reward.

Meaning can organize behavior around something larger than immediate relief. Value-congruent actions—telling the truth, keeping an appointment, taking medication as prescribed, asking for help, apologizing, setting a boundary, or completing a task—may provide evidence from which self-trust can rebuild.

Recovery becomes more durable when life begins to feel worth protecting.

Selected supporting evidence: [57–58,89–90].

Recovery Capital and the Capacity to Use It

Recovery capital is an established construct referring to internal and external resources that may support recovery, including health, housing, family, finances, employment, education, transportation, community, spirituality, and treatment access.

Within the Homeostatic Reserve Model, reserve describes the patient's current functional capacity to recognize, access, tolerate, organize, and use those resources while maintaining regulation. A patient may have substantial resources but be too impaired to use them reliably; another may have strong internal motivation but insufficient housing, treatment, or safety. This distinction is conceptual and has not yet been operationalized against recovery-capital measures.

> *Recovery capital names the resources available; this model focuses on whether the patient can use them under current conditions.*

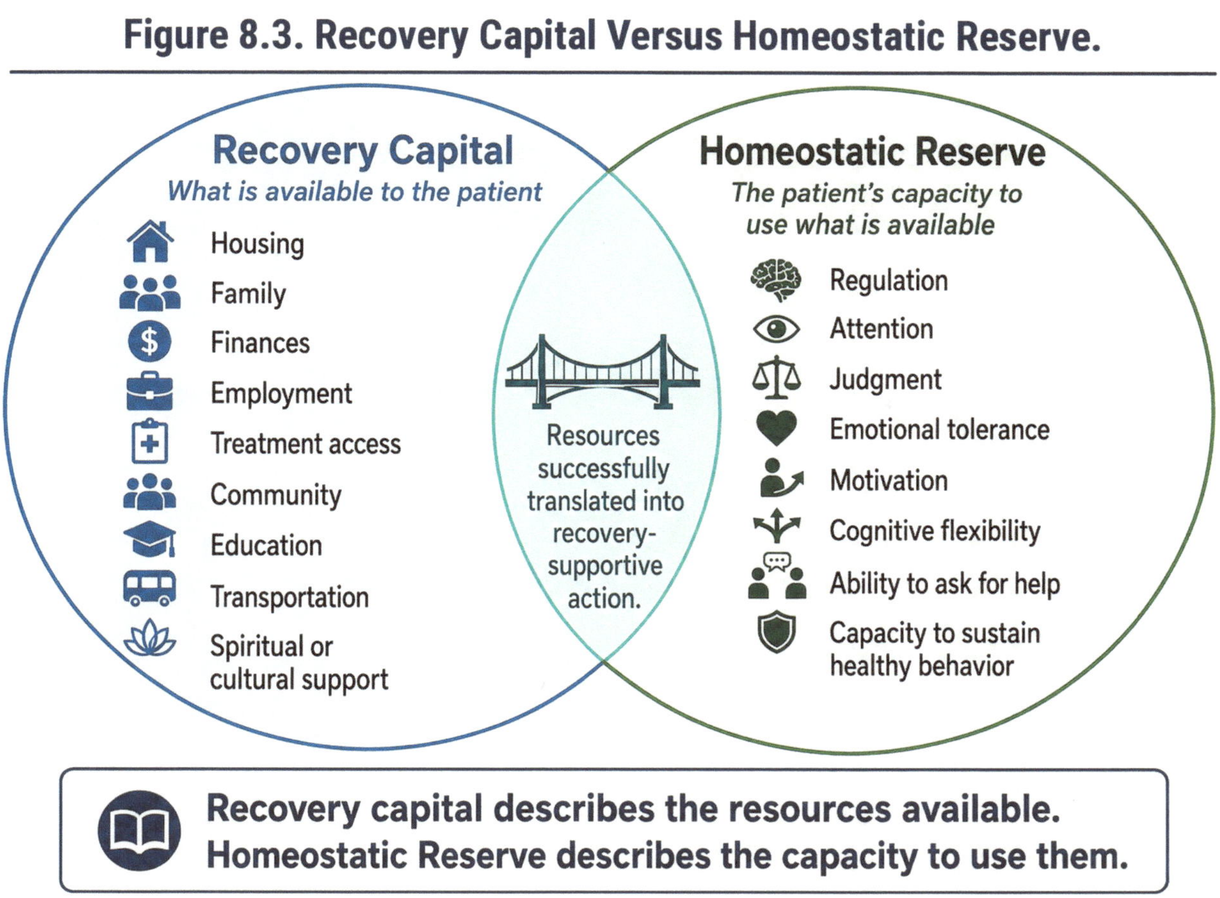

Figure 8.3. Recovery Capital Versus Homeostatic Reserve. Recovery capital includes resources such as housing, family, finances, treatment, community, education, transportation, and work. Within the model, Homeostatic Reserve describes the current capacity to use those resources in recovery-supportive ways. This distinction and figure are conceptual educational representations, not validated cutoff categories or a comparative measurement instrument. Homeostatic Reserve represents integrated regulatory capacity, not a literal dopamine or neurotransmitter supply. Supporting evidence for component mechanisms: [60–62].

Supporting evidence for component mechanisms: [60–62]. These sources support component mechanisms; the model's integrated relationship remains an original conceptual proposition.

Chapter 8 Closing Perspective

Recovery is often built through repeated ordinary actions whose cumulative effect becomes extraordinary.

Chapter 9 moves outward to the environments and resources that can either support this rebuilding or repeatedly overwhelm it.

Chapter Summary

Rebuilding reserve requires coordinated work across biological health, sleep, medication, structure, skills, relationships, natural reward, meaning, and repeated recovery behavior. Recovery is active restoration rather than the passive passage of time.

Key Clinical Takeaways

- Early treatment first addresses major sources of depletion, including withdrawal, medical instability, psychiatric symptoms, sleep disruption, pain, and unsafe access.
- Structure can scaffold behavior from the outside while medication can scaffold regulation from the inside.
- Repetition helps recovery behaviors become more available under stress.
- Recovery capital describes available resources; Homeostatic Reserve describes the person's current capacity to use them.

Chapter 9 — Recovery Capital and the Healing Environment

How External Resources Support Internal Capacity

Recovery does not occur only within the patient. It occurs within a family, home, workplace, treatment system, community, digital environment, and broader social world.

Within the Homeostatic Reserve Model, a patient may work hard to rebuild regulatory capacity and remain vulnerable when the surrounding environment repeatedly creates demands that exceed that capacity. The relationship is conceptual and does not imply a directly measured balance.

> *Recovery is personal, but it is never entirely individual.*

Selected supporting evidence: [57,60–62].

Recovery Capital

Recovery capital is an established construct referring to internal and external resources that can support the initiation and maintenance of recovery. These may include physical and psychiatric health, housing, finances, employment, education, family, transportation, treatment access, recovery community, spirituality, cultural identity, and opportunities for meaningful contribution.

Resources do not guarantee recovery. They must be accessible, usable, and aligned with health. A supportive family may be difficult to use when the patient cannot tolerate feedback. Insurance may exist while the patient cannot organize appointments. Stable housing may contain active use and conflict.

> *Recovery capital describes resources surrounding the patient. Within the model, Homeostatic Reserve describes the current capacity to use them.*

Selected supporting evidence: [60–62].

The Healing Environment

A healing environment is not simply a place where substances are absent. It may reduce avoidable depletion and support repeated recovery-oriented behavior through safety, predictability, structure, care, boundaries, accountability, reduced cue exposure, natural reward, and increasing autonomy. No environment guarantees recovery, and the helpful balance of protection and autonomy varies by patient and phase of care.

> *The purpose of a healing environment is not to eliminate every stressor. It is to reduce avoidable destabilization while the patient builds the capacity to manage ordinary stress.*

Figure 9.1 – Recovery Capital and the Healing Environment

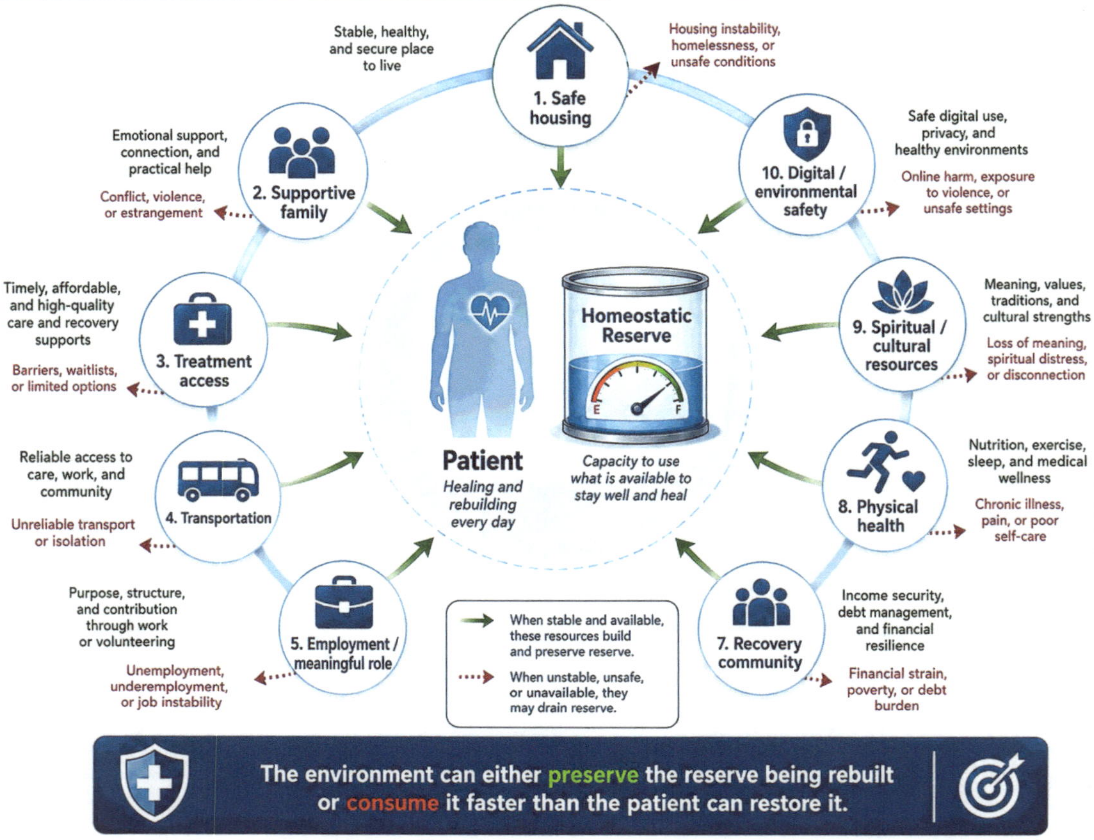

Figure 9.1. Recovery Capital and the Healing Environment. Housing, family, treatment, transportation, finances, work, health, recovery community, culture, spirituality, and digital safety may preserve capacity when stable and recovery-supportive or increase demand when unsafe or unavailable. This figure is a conceptual educational representation, not a validated recovery-capital score, reserve measure, or causal map. Homeostatic Reserve represents integrated regulatory capacity, not a literal dopamine or neurotransmitter supply. Supporting evidence for component mechanisms: [58,60,87–88].

Selected supporting evidence: [58,60,87–88].

Safety Before Growth

A patient worried about where they will sleep, whether they are safe, whether medication is available, how food will be obtained, whether a partner will become violent, or whether substances are present may have less capacity available for reflection, psychotherapy, and long-term planning.

When safety is uncertain, survival demands consume capacity that might otherwise support recovery.

This offers a conceptual parallel to Maslow's hierarchy. Higher-order growth can occur during adversity, and human needs do not unfold as a rigid staircase, but growth may be harder to sustain when the patient repeatedly returns to survival-oriented demands.

Selected supporting evidence: [71,82,87].

Housing, Family, Support, and Boundaries

Stable housing can be an important form of recovery capital because it may support safety, routine, sleep, privacy, medication storage, meals, reduced access, and a base for treatment and work. An address alone is not enough. Housing may remain incompatible with recovery when active use, violence, coercion, conflict, easy access, or absent boundaries are present.

Family and other support systems may provide housing, transport, emotional support, financial help, accountability, encouragement, and continuity. They may also increase demand through conflict, coercion, unsafe surveillance, resentment, unresolved trauma, or patterns that shield ongoing harmful behavior from consequences without increasing treatment, safety, responsibility, or capacity.

> *Family support is most effective when it combines compassion with boundaries.*

Support helps the patient care for the illness. Behaviors sometimes called enabling are better described specifically: reducing an immediate consequence, concealing risk, financing continued use, or repeatedly rescuing without a corresponding increase in treatment, safety, accountability, or capacity.

> *A boundary protects the relationship from becoming organized around the illness.*

Selected supporting evidence: [81,87–88].

Work, Finances, Transportation, and Access

Employment may provide structure, identity, competence, income, social connection, and meaning. It may also drain reserve through excessive hours, sleep disruption, access, trauma exposure, pressure, conflict, or a culture discouraging help-seeking.

Return to work should be matched to current function, treatment needs, and occupational demands rather than time alone. For safety-sensitive professionals, recovery status, treatment level, and fitness for duty remain separate determinations under applicable standards.

Financial stress can intensify shame, anxiety, conflict, and urgency. A problem does not need to be solved immediately before it becomes manageable; it often needs to become organized, understood, and shared.

Transportation and treatment access are easily underestimated. A treatment plan is only as effective as the patient's ability to reach it and use it.

Selected supporting evidence: [57–58,60].

Internal Capacity and External Resources

Within the Homeostatic Reserve Model, internal capacity and external resources are conceptualized as varying partly independently. High reserve and high recovery capital may provide a stronger opportunity for durable recovery; high reserve with limited capital may leave the patient environmentally strained; high capital with low reserve may leave resources difficult to use; and low levels of both may create greater vulnerability. These are descriptive quadrants, not validated cutoffs.

> *Recovery becomes more durable when internal capacity and external resources support the same direction of change.*

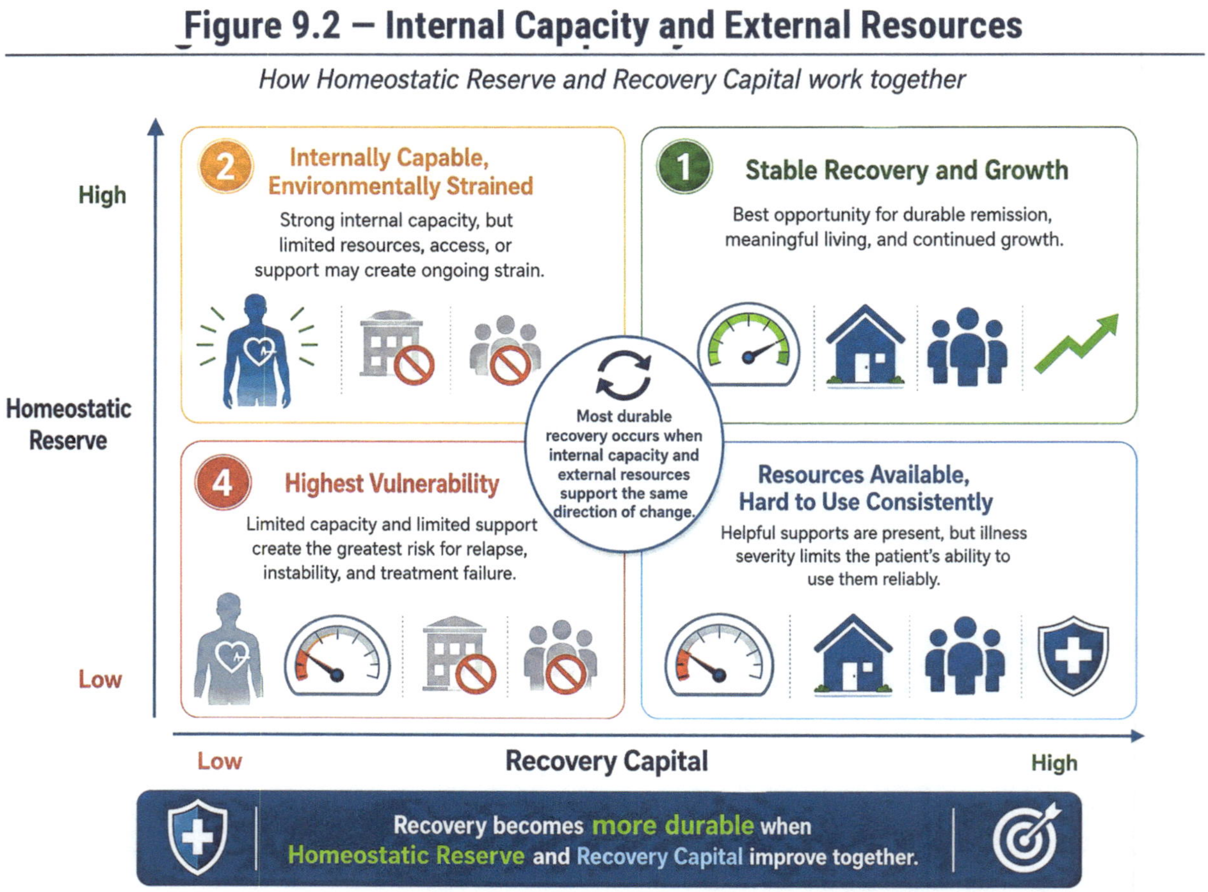

Figure 9.2. Internal Capacity and External Resources. Within the model, recovery may become more durable when Homeostatic Reserve and recovery capital improve together and support the same direction of change. The quadrants are conceptual educational categories, not validated cutoff scores, prognosis groups, or a measurement instrument. Homeostatic Reserve represents integrated regulatory capacity, not a literal dopamine or neurotransmitter supply. Supporting evidence for component mechanisms: [60–62].

Supporting evidence for component mechanisms: [60–62]. These sources support component mechanisms; the model's integrated relationship remains an original conceptual proposition.

Community, Belonging, Peer Support, Culture, and Spirituality

Belonging may reduce isolation and provide identity beyond illness. Recovery communities, peer organizations, faith communities, cultural groups, alumni programs, volunteer work, recreational groups, and healthy friendships may provide connection, hope, ritual, accountability, and meaning. Patients should be offered options that fit their preferences, culture, beliefs, recovery goals, and safety needs.

> *The patient needs more than a place where substances are absent. The patient needs a place where a healthier identity can belong.*

Professional treatment may help explain illness and develop individualized care. Peer support may provide identification, lived-experience knowledge, and repeated opportunities to practice recovery in ordinary life. Neither pathway is identical to or a universal substitute for the other.

Spiritual and cultural resources should neither be imposed nor dismissed. Their clinical value lies in whether they increase connection, humility, meaning, responsibility, and hope.

Selected supporting evidence: [57,66,89–90].

The Digital Environment

The digital environment is an emerging and context-dependent clinical domain. Phones, social media, messaging applications, delivery services, online gambling, and location-based contacts can expose some patients to old networks, cues, conflict, sleep disruption, compulsive behavior, or immediate purchasing access. The same technologies can also support telehealth, meetings, reminders, peer connection, education, and crisis support.

> *The digital environment can function as either recovery capital or a pathway of depletion.*

Selected supporting evidence: [66,86].

Environmental Cues as Neurobiological Stressors

People, places, smells, music, routines, objects, digital contacts, emotional states, and substance availability may activate conditioned memory, salience, stress, craving, and dopamine-linked motivational responses even when no substance is consumed. The magnitude and neural pattern vary by substance, patient, and context.

In some studied populations, human imaging research has demonstrated cue-associated striatal dopamine changes and associations between larger changes and craving. These group-level findings should not be converted into a universal percentage, treated as equivalent to substance exposure, or used to infer an individual patient's dopamine level, receptor status, reserve, or recurrence probability.

> *A substance-related cue may initiate measurable biological, attentional, emotional, and motivational responses; it is not merely a neutral thought about prior use.*

Cue exposure may produce craving, attentional capture, remembered relief, autonomic arousal, narrowed focus, internal conflict, and increased demand on regulation. It is more accurate to describe conditioned motivational and stress activation than literal dopamine depletion.

Selected supporting evidence: [12,25,84–85].

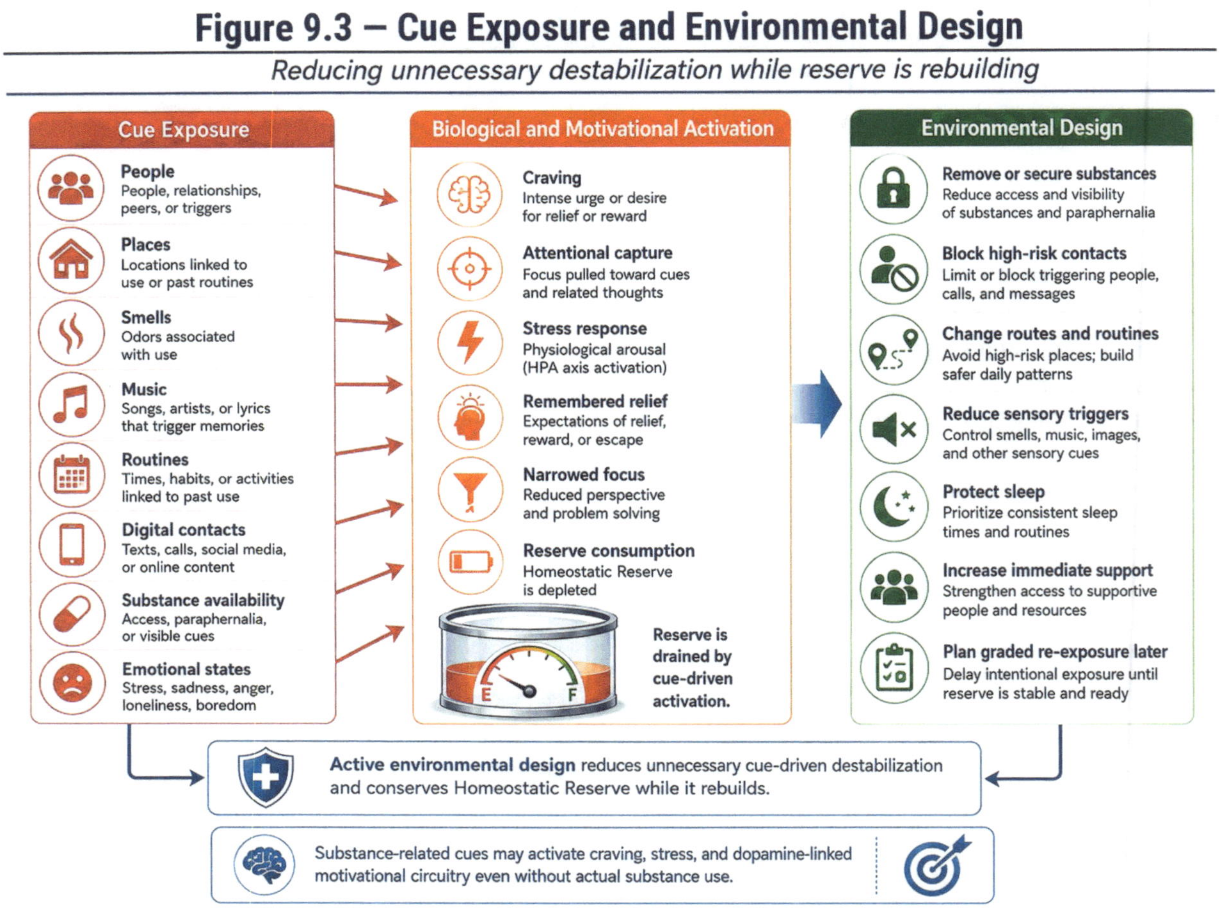

Figure 9.3. Cue Exposure and Environmental Design. Conditioned cues may activate memory, salience, stress, craving, attentional capture, and remembered relief. Individualized environmental design may reduce unnecessary exposure, protect sleep, remove access, change routines, and bring support closer while reserve is rebuilding. This figure is a conceptual educational representation informed by cue-reactivity literature, not a validated cue-response scale, treatment algorithm, or recurrence predictor. Homeostatic Reserve represents integrated regulatory capacity, not a literal dopamine or neurotransmitter supply. Supporting evidence for component mechanisms: [12,25,84–85].

Environmental Design

In early recovery, individualized avoidance of known environmental, social, digital, and sensory triggers may be clinically appropriate. Later work may include planned exposure or broader re-entry when supported by a clear therapeutic rationale, adequate regulation, coping skills, consent, and immediate support. Avoidance and exposure strategies should not be applied as one universal sequence.

Environmental design can be used intentionally to remove or secure substances, block high-risk contacts, change routes and routines, protect sleep, limit money access when clinically and ethically appropriate, and place support closer to moments of vulnerability. The plan should be individualized and revisited as capacity changes.

> *Environmental design can function as an active treatment strategy that reduces avoidable destabilization while capacity is rebuilding.*

> *A patient does not need to prove recovery by remaining unnecessarily close to danger.*

Selected supporting evidence: [69,84,91].

Recovery Capital and the Conditions for Growth

Maslow's hierarchy provides a conceptual, non-rigid parallel. Stable housing, safety, treatment, relationships, meaningful work, and community do not produce recovery automatically. They may reduce survival demands and support connection, competence, meaning, and growth, which can also coexist with adversity.

> *The healing environment does not create human potential. It reduces the conditions that keep that potential trapped in survival.*

Selected supporting evidence: [58,60,62,82].

Chapter 9 Closing Perspective

> *Recovery strengthens when external resources and internal capacity begin to support the same direction of change.*

Chapter 10 turns inward to recognition, acceptance, honesty, and congruence—the processes that allow help to be used and action to align more closely with values.

Chapter Summary

Recovery occurs within an environment. Housing, relationships, work, finances, transportation, access to care, community, digital exposure, and substance-related cues can either support the use of recovery capacity or repeatedly drain it.

Key Clinical Takeaways

- Internal capacity and external resources must be assessed separately and then considered together.
- Supportive environments are protective but not sufficient, and external resources may be difficult to use when reserve is low.
- Cue reactivity can capture attention and increase craving without proving inevitable use.
- Environmental design should be individualized, practical, culturally responsive, and matched to the phase of recovery.

Chapter 10 — Insight, Acceptance, Honesty, and Congruence

How Recognition Becomes Recovery-Oriented Action

Addictive illness may impair the patient's ability to recognize the illness, tolerate what recognition means, and organize life around care. A patient may stop using without understanding the illness, comply without accepting necessity, or acknowledge consequences while believing the larger pattern does not apply. These presentations should be distinguished from ordinary defense, shame, ambivalence, incomplete memory, cultural context, and intentional concealment.

> *Recognition means seeing the evidence. Acceptance means allowing the evidence to change how one lives.*

Selected supporting evidence: [31,69–70].

Denial as Human Response and Illness-Related Impairment

Denial is not unique to addiction. A patient may resist diabetes, hypertension, cancer, bipolar disorder, psychosis, cognitive decline, or another serious diagnosis because it threatens identity, independence, role, self-esteem, and the anticipated future.

Addictive illness may add the complication that brain systems involved in salience, self-monitoring, memory, emotional tolerance, and executive control are affected while the substance remains a rapidly available source of relief. This can strengthen minimization or resistance in some patients but does not create one universal form of denial.

> *Denial may begin as a human defense. In addictive illness it may also be strengthened by impaired insight, altered salience, memory limitations, shame, ambivalence, or the learned value of immediate relief.*

Selected supporting evidence: [31,33,69].

Recognition Is Not Acceptance

Within the Homeostatic Reserve Model, recognition describes seeing relevant evidence, while acceptance describes allowing that evidence to alter care and behavior. A patient may recognize withdrawal, family conflict, occupational problems, medical consequences, failed attempts to stop, or recurrence while explaining each event separately.

> *The patient may recognize every consequence separately while remaining unable to recognize the illness connecting them.*

Repeated consequences may weaken explanations that protect denial, but treatment should not wait for the patient to accumulate enough suffering to hit bottom.

Within this clinical framework, acceptance is not surrender of hope or identity. It is the developing willingness to recognize that an illness is present and organize life in a way that takes it seriously. Recognition and acceptance are useful conceptual distinctions, not validated stages or biomarkers.

> *Acceptance is not giving up. It is stopping the argument with reality long enough to begin caring for the illness.*

Selected supporting evidence: [31,69–70].

Acceptance May Deepen Over Time

Acceptance is rarely one moment and does not follow one required sequence. A patient may gradually accept that use has become dangerous, that willpower alone has not been sufficient, that treatment must be stronger or longer, or that medication, structure, monitoring, or community support may be helpful. Different aspects may develop, coexist, advance, or recede over time.

> *Acceptance becomes clinically meaningful when it changes what the patient is willing to do.*

Acceptance can reduce the emotional and cognitive energy spent explaining consequences, defending prior decisions, concealing symptoms, bargaining about treatment, and proving independence.

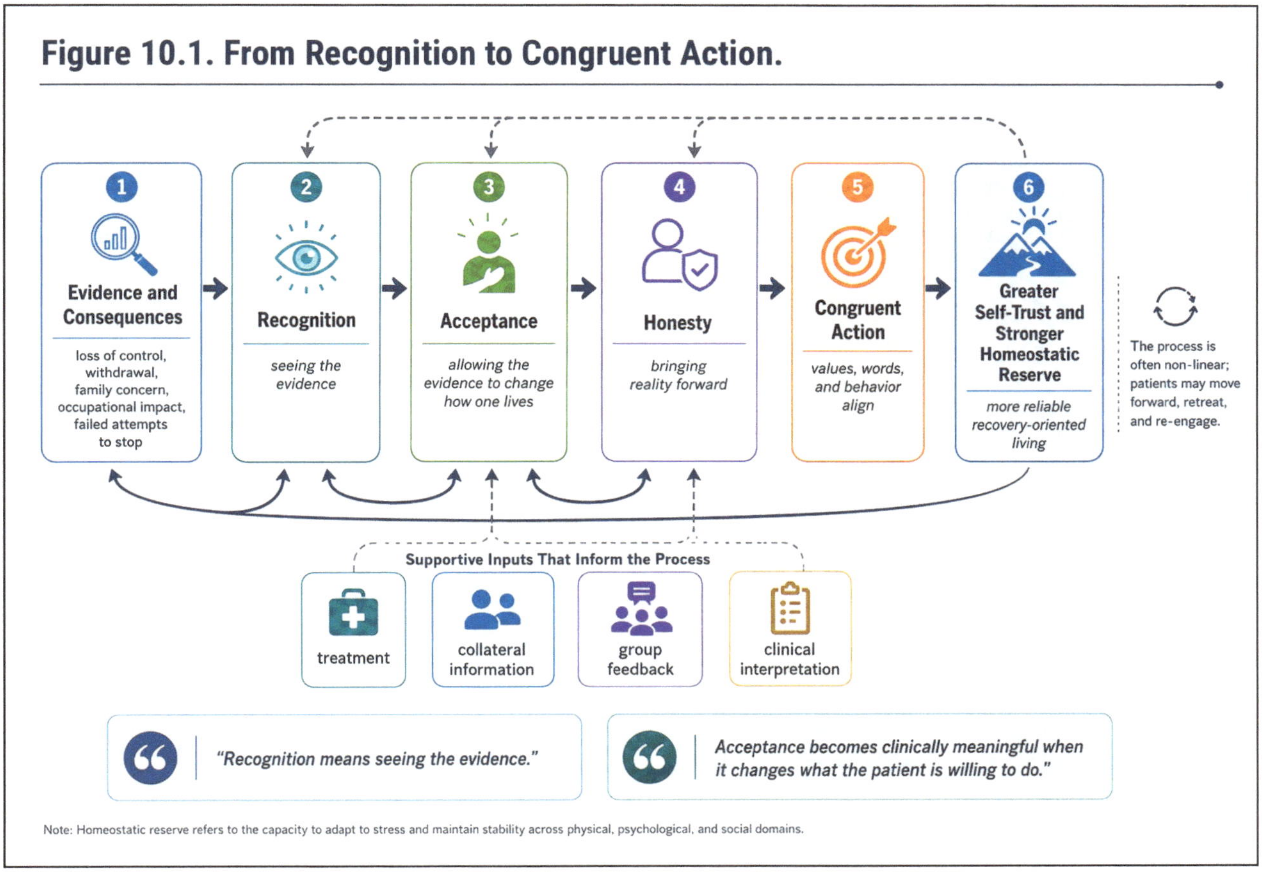

Figure 10.1. From Recognition to Congruent Action. Within the model, evidence and consequences may contribute to recognition, acceptance, recovery-relevant honesty, congruent action, greater self-trust, and stronger reserve. The path is nonlinear and may require repeated feedback and re-engagement. This figure is a conceptual educational representation, not a validated stage model, biomarker, or measurement instrument. Homeostatic Reserve represents integrated regulatory capacity, not a literal dopamine or neurotransmitter supply. Supporting evidence for component mechanisms: [31,69–70].

Selected supporting evidence: [69–70].

Honesty as a Developing Recovery Capacity

Patients entering treatment may not yet disclose the illness fully. They may minimize, omit, distort, or compartmentalize because of fear, shame, impaired insight, cognitive disruption, concern about consequences, attachment to the substance, intentional concealment, or uncertainty about whether treatment is safe enough for disclosure.

Families, patients, and treatment teams may expect immediate total disclosure. When it does not occur, they may conclude that treatment is failing. Within the Homeostatic Reserve Model, increasing recovery-relevant honesty is conceptualized as one capacity treatment may strengthen. It is not a biological marker, validated stage, or stand-alone measure of recovery.

The patient may initially disclose only what can no longer be denied. Later, they may acknowledge additional consequences, craving, ambivalence, medication misuse, recurrence-related thinking, resentment, fear, and earlier behaviors.

The clinical importance of honesty remains high, while expectations for perfect early performance should remain realistic. Observable recovery-relevant behaviors may include correcting an earlier account without being confronted, disclosing craving before acting, acknowledging ambivalence, reporting loss of routine, identifying minimization, or asking for help before crisis. These behaviors are clinical observations, not a validated honesty score or biomarker.

The goal is not a claim of perfect honesty. It is increasingly reliable disclosure of clinically meaningful vulnerability.

> *Honesty begins as something treatment asks of the patient and gradually becomes something the patient uses to protect recovery.*

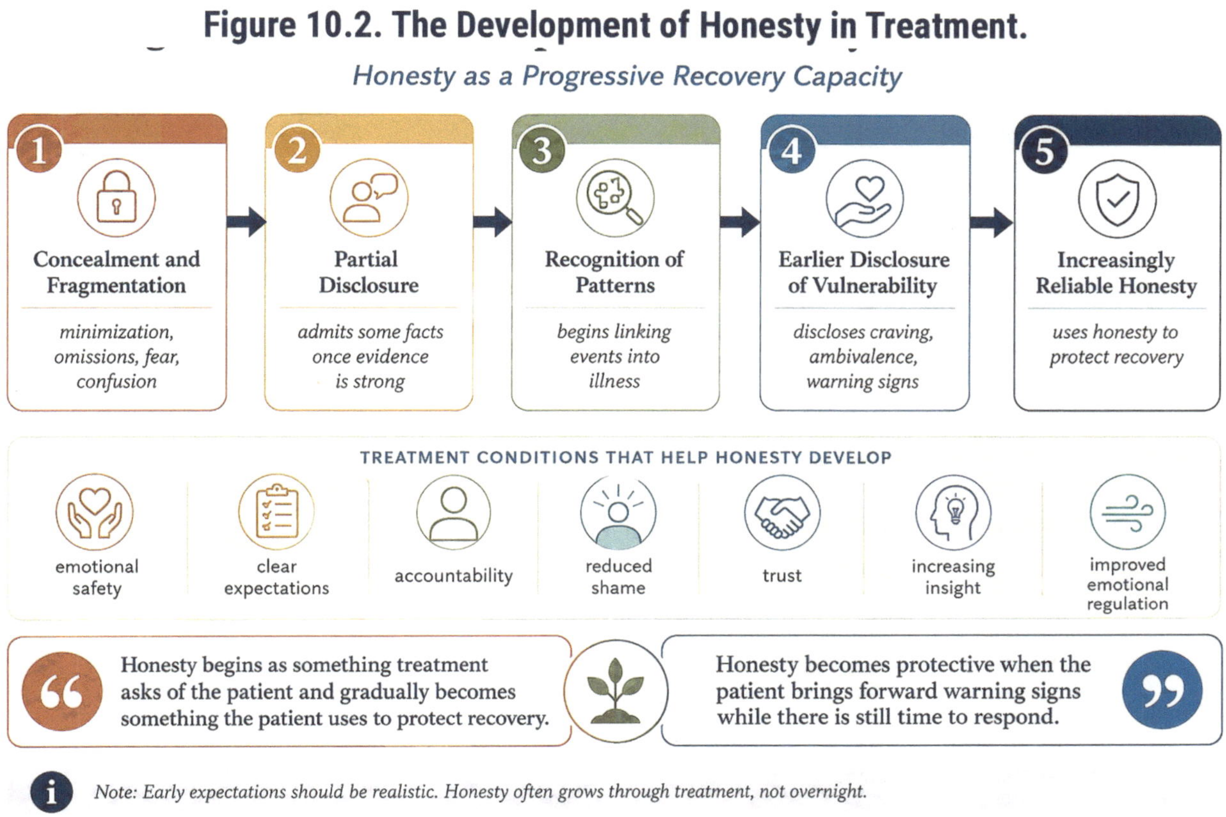

Figure 10.2. The Development of Recovery-Relevant Honesty. Honesty may move from concealment and fragmentation toward partial disclosure, recognition of patterns, earlier disclosure of vulnerability, and increasingly reliable recovery-oriented communication. This is a conceptual educational representation, not a validated staging system, biomarker, or measure of moral worth. Homeostatic Reserve represents integrated regulatory capacity, not a literal dopamine or neurotransmitter supply. Supporting evidence for component mechanisms: [65,69,91].

Selected supporting evidence: [65,69,91].

Honesty, Privacy, and the Treatment Environment

Honesty is more than confession. It may include reporting craving, fantasies of use, worsening sleep, emotional instability, cue exposure, medication misuse, isolation, resentment, and loss of recovery routines. Not every thought must be shared with every person. Healthy privacy remains important, and disclosure should follow informed consent, confidentiality, mandatory-reporting, safety, monitoring, and other applicable legal and ethical boundaries.

> *Honesty is not the abandonment of privacy. It is the refusal to let secrecy protect the illness.*

Honesty is more likely to deepen in an environment combining clear expectations, emotional safety, consistency, confidentiality within appropriate limits, accountability, respect, and freedom from humiliation. Collateral communication and disclosure should use patient authorization or another valid legal basis except when safety or law requires otherwise.

> *The patient is more likely to tell the truth when the truth is met with seriousness, clarity, and care rather than humiliation.*

Selected supporting evidence: [65,69,81].

Congruence and Self-Respect

Within the Homeostatic Reserve Model, congruence refers to the increasing alignment of thoughts, words, values, and actions. Early recovery may contain substantial incongruence. A patient may sincerely want recovery while engaging in behaviors that serve the illness because reserve, insight, skill, support, or willingness remains limited. Congruence is a clinical proposition and teaching construct, not a biomarker or validated score.

> *Congruence is the gradual recovery of alignment between values and action.*

Incongruent behavior may contribute to guilt, shame, secrecy, anxiety, conflict, and loss of self-trust; these states may increase demand on regulation and intensify relief seeking. Value-congruent action may support self-respect, willingness to protect oneself, stronger reserve, and further congruent action. Within the model, this is a proposed reciprocal relationship, not a demonstrated linear causal law.

> *Self-trust is rebuilt through repeated evidence.*

A useful patient-facing formulation is: "When I feel good about me, it becomes easier to treat me well." Often the healthier action comes first and gradually changes how the patient feels about themselves.

Selected supporting evidence: [58,69,89].

External and Internal Motivation

Patients may begin treatment because of family pressure, professional monitoring, employment requirements, legal consequences, medical danger, loss of housing, or fear of losing a relationship. External motivation is clinically meaningful because it can create safety and time for engagement. External and internal motives can coexist throughout recovery.

As treatment progresses, the patient may understand the illness personally: the loss of freedom, repeated consequences, limits of private control, effect on loved ones, and danger of returning to prior behavior.

> *External motivation may bring the patient into treatment. Growing insight, acceptance, connection, hope, and self-respect may help reasons for recovery become increasingly personal, but this is not a required one-way sequence.*

Jerry Gropper, DDS, LP, CAP, in A Guide to Growing Up—Addiction Recovery, captured a motivational turning point in recovery with this teaching phrase:

> *"Fear of the Disease becomes greater than Fear of Change." [100]*

Within the Homeostatic Reserve Model, the phrase describes a shift in salience: fear of continuing the illness can become strong enough to open the door to change, while hope, meaning, connection, and restored freedom help make recovery increasingly internal and sustainable.

Figure 10.3. From External to Internal Motivation.

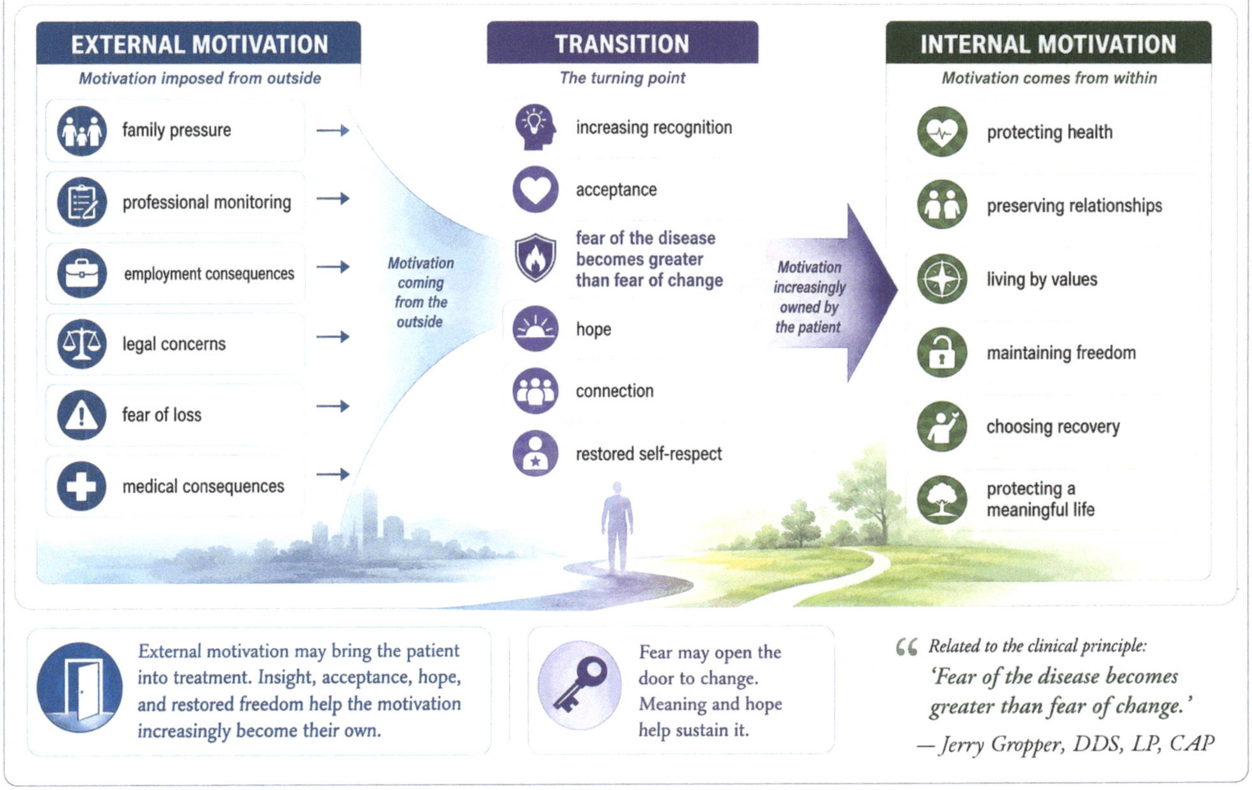

Figure 10.3. From External Toward More Internalized Motivation. External pressure may initiate treatment, while recognition, acceptance, hope, connection, and restored self-respect may help motivation become increasingly personal. External and internal motives may coexist, and the trajectory is not universal. The teaching phrase "Fear of the Disease becomes greater than Fear of Change," attributed to Jerry Gropper, DDS, LP, CAP, is used as a concise clinical formulation of one possible motivational turning point. This figure is a conceptual educational representation, not a validated stage model or motivation scale. Homeostatic Reserve represents integrated regulatory capacity, not a literal dopamine or neurotransmitter supply. Supporting evidence for component mechanisms and attribution: [69–70,100].

Selected supporting evidence and attribution: [69–70,100].

Collateral Information, Group Recognition, and Collaborative Feedback

Memory and self-observation may be incomplete. Collateral information from family, employers, prior clinicians, records, and monitoring programs may become part of the diagnostic mirror when obtained with patient authorization or another valid legal or ethical basis. The need for collateral must be balanced with privacy, therapeutic alliance, safety, mandatory reporting, and occupation-specific monitoring requirements.

When self-observation is impaired, the observations of others may become part of the diagnostic mirror.

Groups can be powerful because patients may recognize patterns in others before recognizing similar patterns in themselves. Feedback and discrepancy-focused intervention have a role when they are collaborative, specific, evidence-based, respectful, proportionate, non-shaming, and connected to treatment goals. Coercive or humiliating confrontation can undermine safety and engagement.

> *The purpose of feedback is not to win an argument. It is to make a discrepancy visible enough that the patient can examine and respond to it.*

Selected supporting evidence: [65,69,81].

How Insight Becomes Protective Capacity

Recognition may reduce fragmentation; acceptance may direct effort toward care; honesty may give treatment access to reality; congruence may reduce internal conflict; and more personal motivation may support sustained action. Within the model, these processes may strengthen functional capacity, but the integrated pathway has not been validated as a composite mechanism.

When regulation deteriorates, defensiveness, secrecy, and survival-oriented behavior may return. The clinical response is earlier assessment, restored support, and clear attention to safety and accountability—not moral condemnation.

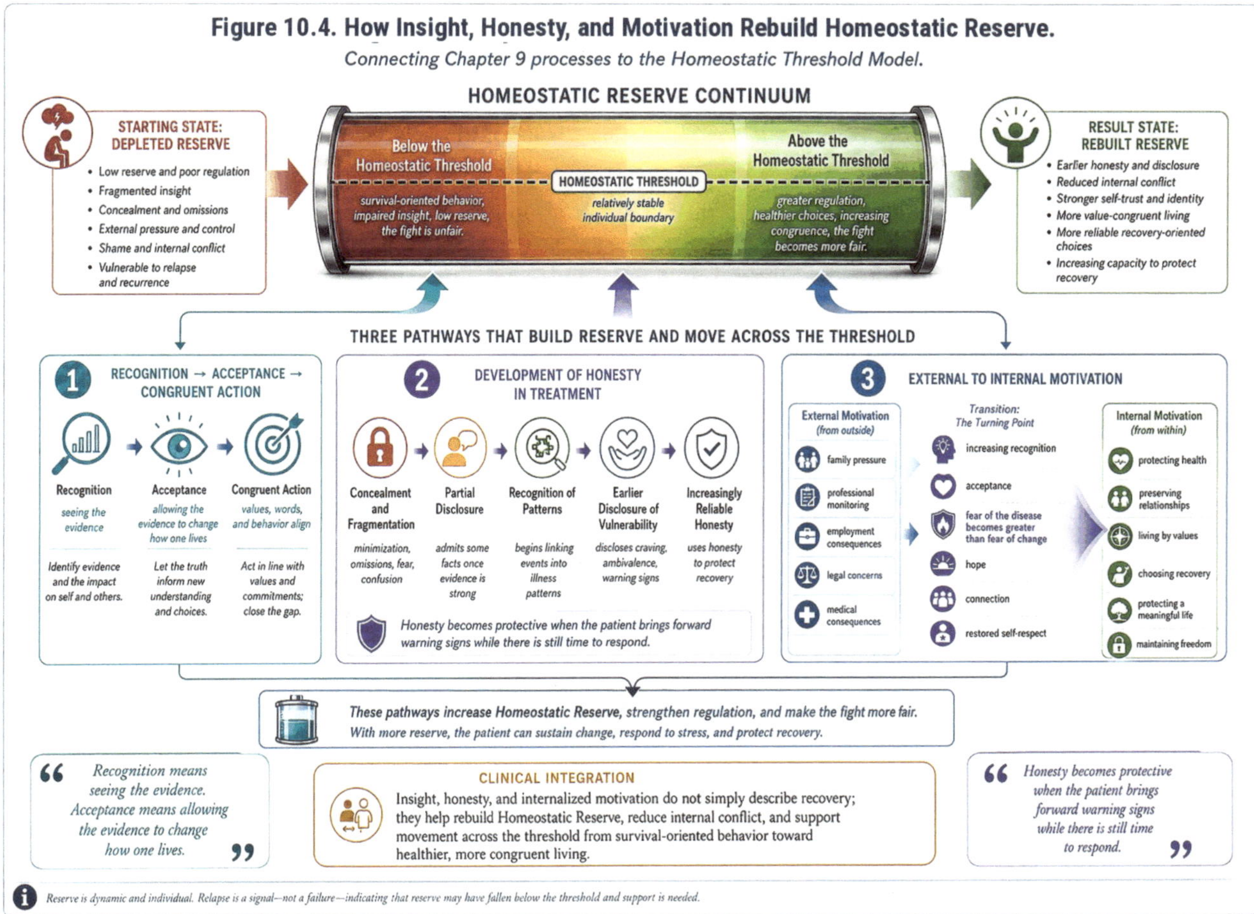

Figure 10.4. Homeostatic Reserve and Pathways to Recovery. Within the model, recognition, acceptance, honesty, congruent action, and internalized motivation interact with reserve and the conceptual threshold. When reserve falls, defensiveness and survival-oriented behavior may increase; when reserve rebuilds, values, support, and healthier action may become more available. This figure is a conceptual educational representation, not a validated causal pathway, stage model, biomarker, or measurement instrument. Homeostatic Reserve represents integrated regulatory capacity, not a literal dopamine or neurotransmitter supply. Supporting evidence for component mechanisms: [31,58,69].

Chapter 10 Closing Perspective

Honesty makes vulnerability visible early enough for treatment and support to act.

Chapter 11 applies these capacities to the daily work of protecting remission before vulnerability becomes crisis.

Chapter Summary

Insight, acceptance, honesty, and congruence are developing clinical capacities rather than binary traits or biomarkers. They are influenced by cognitive function, shame, fear, safety, memory, consequences, relationships, and the person's ability to tolerate what recognition means.

Key Clinical Takeaways

- Denial is not one phenomenon; it may include defense, impaired insight, ambivalence, memory limitations, shame, or intentional concealment.
- Recognition does not automatically produce acceptance or sustained behavioral change.
- Recovery-relevant honesty means increasingly reliable disclosure of information that affects safety and treatment, not the elimination of all privacy.
- Collaborative feedback and collateral information should be accurate, respectful, legally appropriate, and non-humiliating.

Chapter 11 — Protecting Remission and Maintaining Recovery

How Patients Recognize Vulnerability Early and Respond Before Recurrence

Recovery is not protected by one decision made at discharge. It is protected through repeated decisions made before vulnerability becomes crisis.

A patient may complete treatment with stronger regulatory capacity, improved regulation, meaningful insight, and more internalized motivation. Within the model, that capacity remains dynamic. Sleep loss, illness, grief, conflict, cue exposure, isolation, pain, psychiatric symptoms, work pressure, and loss of structure may increase demand; the effect of any factor varies by patient and context.

> *Recovery is protected most effectively before the patient feels close to recurrence.*

Selected supporting evidence: [63–64,91].

Remission Is a Living Condition

Within the Homeostatic Reserve Model, remission is conceptualized as an actively supported condition rather than a static possession. Sleep, indicated medication, honest relationships, recovery activity, manageable stress, healthy routines, and access to care may help protect it. When several supports weaken together, vulnerability may increase even when the patient remains committed to recovery.

> *A patient can remain committed to recovery while becoming biologically and psychologically less able to protect it.*

Changes Often Precede Substance Use

Return to use is often preceded by detectable changes such as worsening sleep, irritability, reduced treatment attendance, isolation, romanticizing prior use, secrecy, medication nonadherence, resentment toward recovery demands, renewed contact with high-risk people, reduced natural reward, or overconfidence. Not every recurrence follows the same sequence, and some episodes occur despite substantial planning and support.

A warning sign is not always the cause. Poor sleep may be a warning sign, contributing factor, or both. The goal is to notice meaningful deviation from the patient's stable recovery pattern.

> *Warning signs are most useful when interpreted in the context of the patient's own stable pattern.*

Risk Accumulates Before Crisis

A patient may tolerate one night of poor sleep, one conflict, one missed appointment, or one unexpected cue. When poor sleep, conflict, pain, isolation, and cue exposure occur together, cumulative demand may exceed current capacity. This accumulation is individualized and is not represented by a numerical reserve score.

> *Recurrence risk often rises through accumulation rather than one isolated cause.*

As cumulative demand grows, thinking may narrow, urgency may rise, frustration tolerance may fall, cue reactivity may increase, and willingness to seek help may decline. These changes are clinically important but do not constitute a validated recurrence predictor.

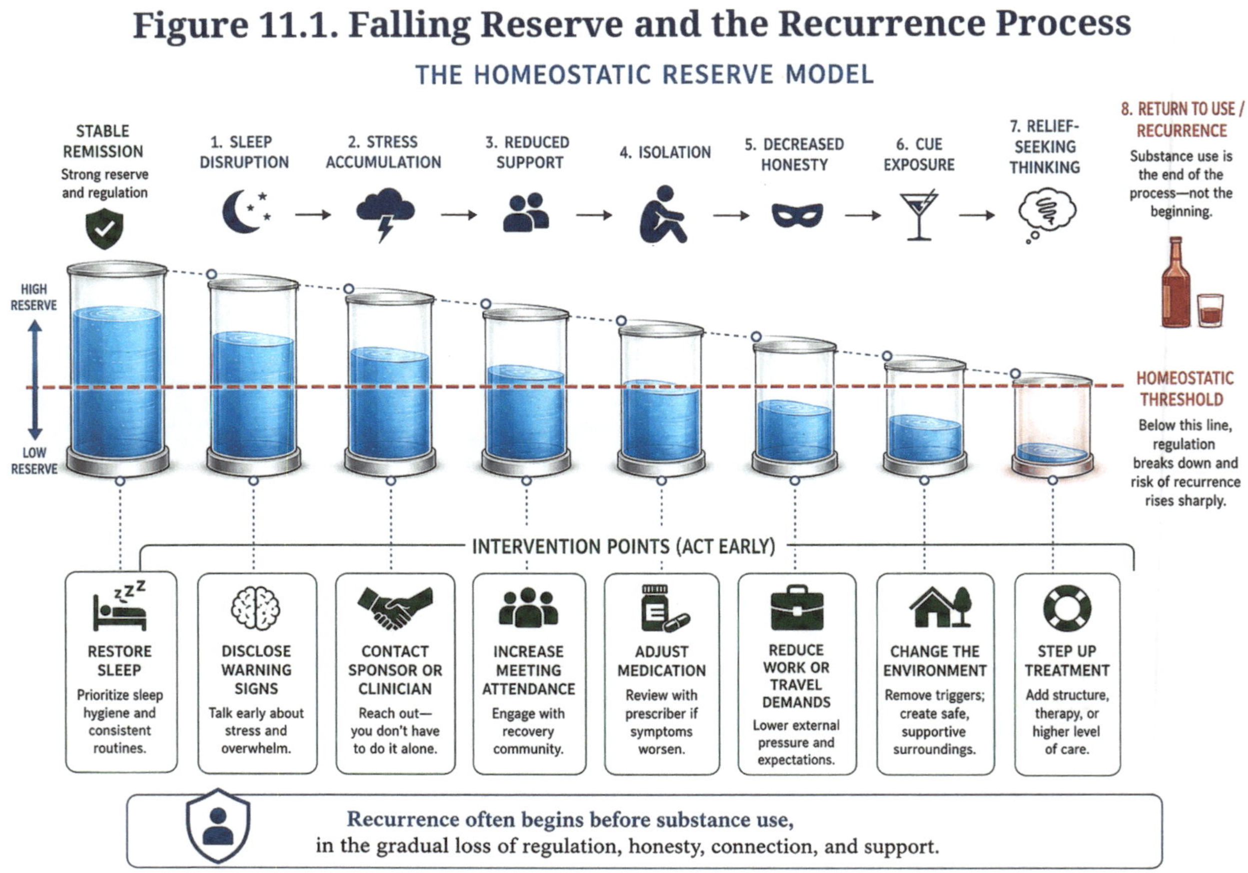

Figure 11.1. Falling Reserve and the Recurrence Process. Sleep disruption, cumulative stress, reduced support, isolation, decreasing honesty, cue exposure, and relief-seeking thinking may increase vulnerability before substance use occurs, while multiple early intervention points may remain available. This figure is a conceptual educational representation, not a validated recurrence sequence, risk calculator, or prediction instrument. Homeostatic Reserve represents integrated regulatory capacity, not a literal dopamine or neurotransmitter supply. Supporting evidence for component mechanisms: [25,55,63,91].

A Specific Early Response Plan

A general instruction to call someone if things become bad is often insufficient. An individualized plan may identify the patient's earliest warning signs, who should be contacted, which clinician will respond, what support persons should do, when medication should be reviewed, when work or travel should be reduced, and what findings require urgent evaluation or a higher level of care.

The plan should tell the patient what to do before judgment becomes significantly impaired.

The plan should be created while the patient is stable enough to participate thoughtfully and should be simple enough to use when cognition and motivation are narrowing.

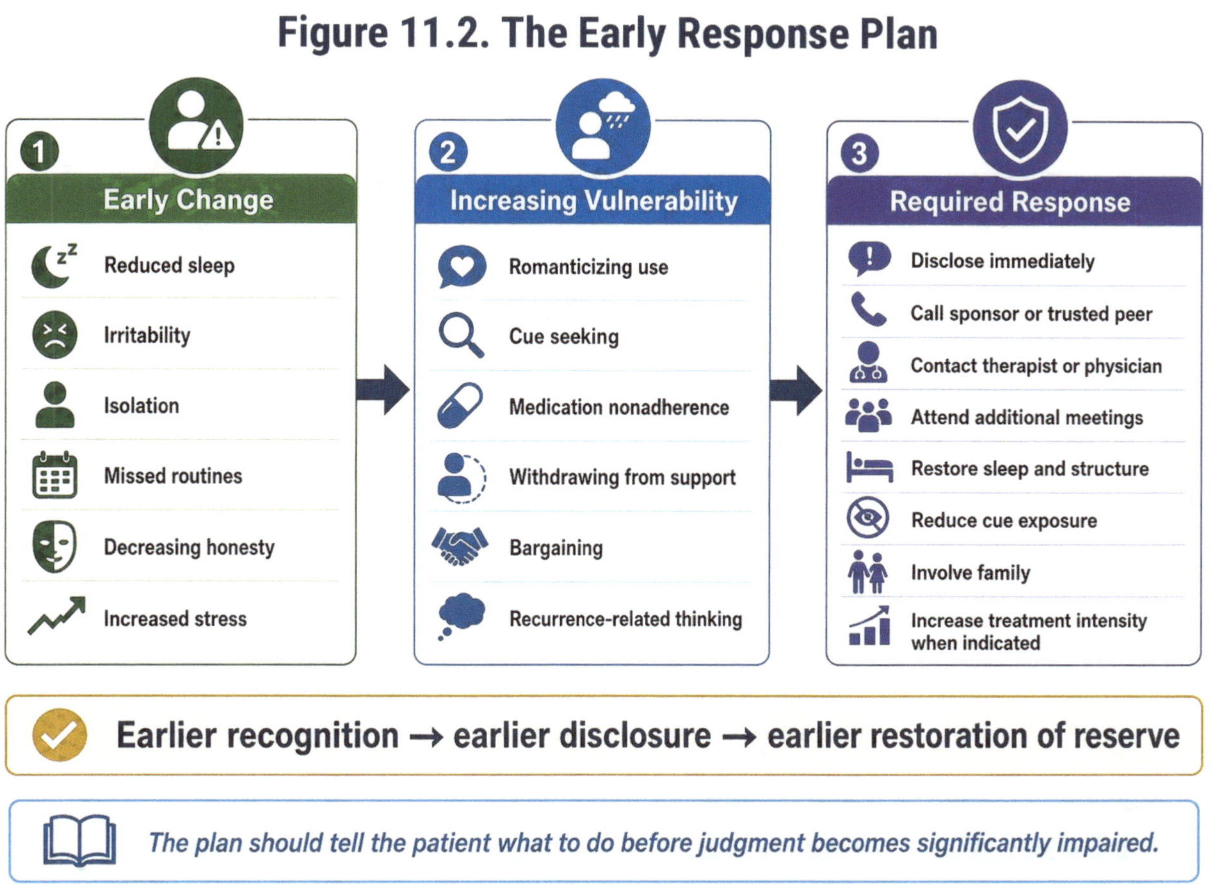

Figure 11.2. The Early Response Plan. Individualized early changes and increasing vulnerability may trigger disclosure, peer or sponsor contact when relevant, clinical contact, additional meetings, restoration of sleep and structure, cue reduction, support-system involvement, and increased treatment intensity when indicated. This figure is a conceptual educational representation, not a validated universal protocol, decision rule, or level-of-care algorithm. Homeostatic Reserve represents integrated regulatory capacity, not a literal dopamine or neurotransmitter supply. Supporting evidence for component mechanisms: [63,69,91].

Honesty as an Early Intervention

The patient may notice craving, loss of interest in recovery, resentment, fantasies of controlled use, medication misuse, renewed contact with high-risk people, or fear of disappointing the team. The safest response is to bring information forward early.

> *Honesty becomes protective when the patient brings forward warning signs while there is still time to respond.*

Early disclosure may allow increased visits, medication adjustment, return to group, temporary reduction in work demand, restoration of sleep, environmental change, family involvement, or transition to a higher level of care.

Selected supporting evidence: [69,91].

A Return to Support Is Not Failure

Patients may resist stepping up care because of embarrassment, fear of losing independence, occupational consequences, family disappointment, or the belief that increased treatment proves recovery has failed.

> *Returning to support is not evidence that recovery failed. It is evidence that the patient is using recovery to respond to changing need.*

A patient with diabetes may need medication adjustment during illness. A person with asthma may need more intensive care during an exacerbation. A person in recovery may need temporary intensification when vulnerability rises.

Community Support Meetings, Sponsorship, and Learning How to Live

Many patients benefit from support beyond scheduled appointments with a therapist or physician. Mutual-support meetings and other recovery communities may provide frequent contact, identification, accountability, practical guidance, hope, continuity, and a place to discuss vulnerability before crisis. Patients should be offered evidence-informed options that fit their diagnosis, goals, culture, beliefs, preferences, and safety needs.

Some patients describe community support as helping them learn how to live. Professional treatment may help the patient understand illness, regulate symptoms, process trauma or grief, and develop a plan. Mutual support may provide repeated opportunities to practice honesty, humility, responsibility, relationship skills, service, and recovery-oriented decision-making in ordinary life. Neither is a universal substitute for the other.

> *Treatment helps the patient understand the illness. A recovery community can help the patient practice how to live with that understanding every day.*

Alcoholics Anonymous and Twelve-Step Facilitation

Alcoholics Anonymous is a voluntary, peer-led mutual-help fellowship for people seeking recovery from alcohol problems. Twelve-Step Facilitation is a distinct, professionally delivered, structured intervention designed to increase engagement with AA or related Twelve-Step mutual-help practices. They should not be treated as interchangeable terms.

For alcohol use disorder, a 2020 Cochrane review found that manualized AA/Twelve-Step Facilitation interventions improved continuous abstinence compared with some established treatments and may reduce healthcare costs, while many other alcohol-related outcomes were generally comparable. These findings should not be generalized automatically to every AA meeting, every nonmanualized Twelve-Step program, all substance-use disorders, or every patient. Secular, cultural, faith-based, and other mutual-support pathways may also be appropriate.

> *For many people with alcohol use disorder, AA is an evidence-supported mutual-help pathway; Twelve-Step Facilitation is a separate professional intervention that can help patients engage with it.*

Selected supporting evidence: [63–64,91].

The Role of a Sponsor

A sponsor is a nonprofessional peer within a Twelve-Step fellowship. Roles and practices vary. A sponsor is not a physician, therapist, addiction counselor, case manager, or emergency clinician; should not diagnose, prescribe, direct medication changes, provide emergency care, or replace licensed professional treatment; and should encourage clinical or emergency contact when risk exceeds the peer role. A sponsor may help with

Steps, meeting engagement, identification, rationalization, ordinary frustration, honesty, service, and seeking help before isolation deepens.

> *A sponsor may provide trusted, recovery-informed peer guidance between clinical appointments and ordinary daily decisions.*

A trusted sponsor or community member may be helpful when resentment, isolation, romanticizing use, avoidance of meetings, or other warning signs appear. The patient should also have multiple pathways to professional and emergency care, including clinicians, family or other support persons, peers, crisis services, and emergency resources.

Meetings, Step Work, and Service as Recovery Practices

Within the Homeostatic Reserve Model, meetings, sponsorship, step work, service, and trusted recovery relationships may strengthen functional capacity through connection, regulation, meaning, honesty, accountability, hope, belonging, recovery identity, and successful coping. “Filling the tank” remains teaching language, not a measured biological process.

A meeting may reduce isolation. A sponsor may organize a confusing moment. Step work may reduce shame and internal conflict. Service may strengthen meaning and identity.

The Recovery Maintenance Network

Within the Homeostatic Reserve Model, the Recovery Maintenance Network is a conceptual synthesis of complementary supports. Depending on the patient, a physician may address biological, psychiatric, medical, and medication-related change; a therapist may address emotion, trauma, grief, and relationships; an addiction counselor may address daily recovery behavior and accountability; sponsors and peers may provide identification and community; family or other support persons may provide observation, support, and boundaries; and monitoring or structured treatment may add protection. No single configuration is required for every patient.

> *The safest recovery plan provides more than one person to call and more than one pathway back toward regulation.*

Figure 11.3. The Recovery Maintenance Network

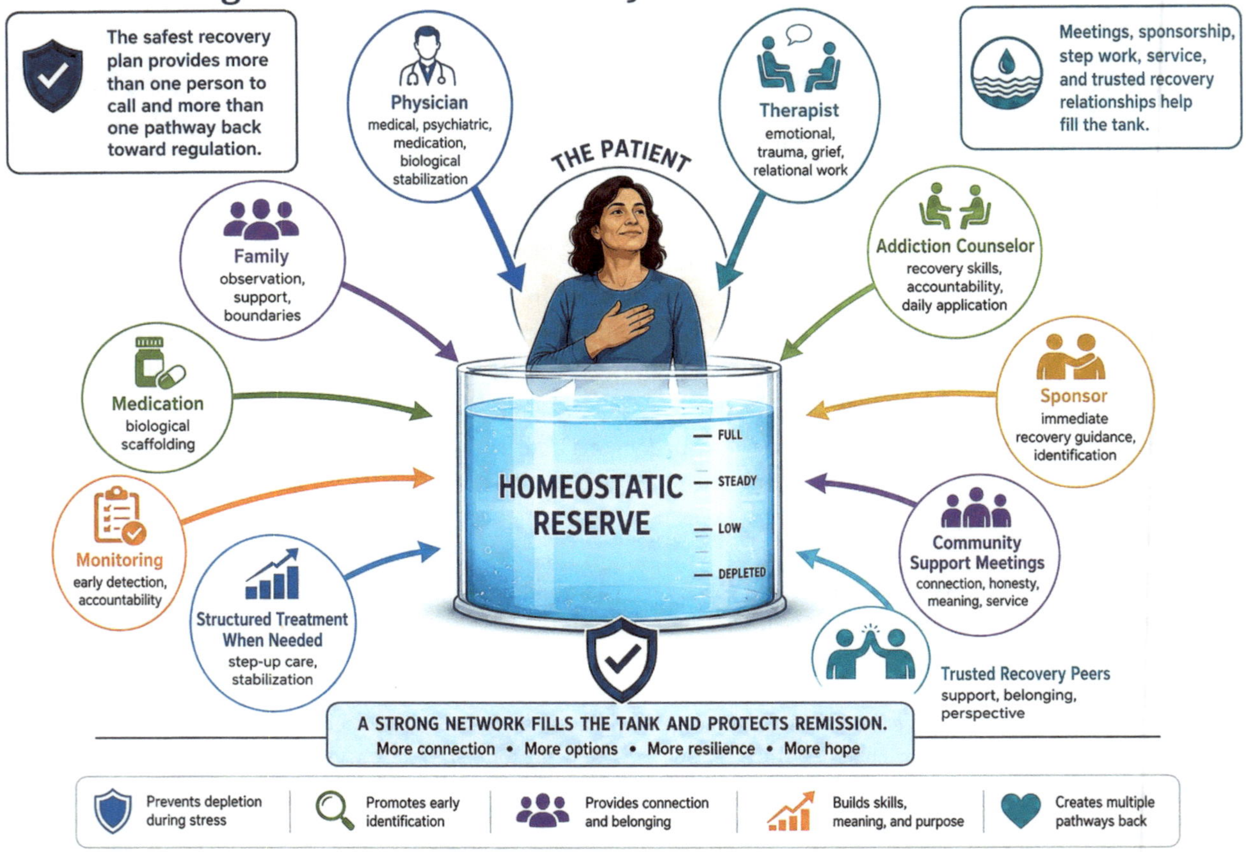
The safest recovery plan provides more than one person to call and more than one pathway back toward regulation.
Physician
medical, psychiatric, medication, biological stabilization
THE PATIENT
Therapist
emotional, trauma, grief, relational work
Meetings, sponsorship, step work, service, and trusted recovery relationships help fill the tank.
Family
observation, support, boundaries
Addiction Counselor
recovery skills, accountability, daily application
Medication
biological scaffolding
Sponsor
immediate recovery guidance, identification
HOMEOSTATIC RESERVE
FULL
STEADY
LOW
DEPLETED
Monitoring
early detection, accountability
Community Support Meetings
connection, honesty, meaning, service
Structured Treatment When Needed
step-up care, stabilization
Trusted Recovery Peers
support, belonging, perspective
A STRONG NETWORK FILLS THE TANK AND PROTECTS REMISSION.
More connection • More options • More resilience • More hope
Prevents depletion during stress
Promotes early identification
Provides connection and belonging
Builds skills, meaning, and purpose
Creates multiple pathways back

Figure 11.3. The Recovery Maintenance Network. Physicians, therapists, addiction counselors, sponsors, community meetings, peers, family or other support persons, medication, monitoring, and structured treatment are shown as possible complementary pathways that may protect remission and support reserve. This figure is an original conceptual educational synthesis, not a validated care plan, required network, or level-of-care instrument. Homeostatic Reserve represents integrated regulatory capacity, not a literal dopamine or neurotransmitter supply. Supporting evidence for component mechanisms: [36,63,65–67].

Supporting evidence for component mechanisms: [36,63,65–68,93]. These sources support component mechanisms; the model's integrated relationship remains an original conceptual proposition.

Medication, Monitoring, Sleep, Stress, and Cue Exposure

Indicated medication may continue during remission. Feeling better can reflect treatment effectiveness and is not, by itself, evidence that medication should stop. Continuation, adjustment, or discontinuation should follow diagnosis- and medication-specific evidence, response, adverse effects, patient preference, recurrence history, psychiatric and medical stability, occupational considerations, and available support—not a predetermined duration or reserve estimate.

Monitoring may include clinical visits, toxicology, medication counts, prescription-monitoring review, authorized family feedback, workplace reports when legally and ethically appropriate, peer contact, digital safeguards, or professional monitoring programs. The type, frequency, duration, confidentiality boundaries, and response plan should be individualized and consistent with consent, law, occupation-specific standards, and clinical need.

Monitoring does not replace recovery. It helps detect change while recovery is still protectable.

Sleep disturbance can be an important early warning sign for some patients, who may benefit from a plan for several nights of deterioration rather than waiting for exhaustion. Cumulative stress matters even when no single dramatic event occurs. Unexpected cue exposure may prompt leaving the setting, contacting support, discussing the reaction honestly, restoring sleep and routine, and increasing care when clinically indicated; responses should be individualized.

Recovery does not require proving strength by standing close to danger.

Overconfidence, Stability, and Accurate Respect

Improvement can paradoxically increase vulnerability. As the patient feels better, prior severity becomes less emotionally vivid. They may believe treatment was excessive, monitoring is unnecessary, support is for less stable people, or controlled use is now possible.

Recovery can become vulnerable when improvement is mistaken for immunity.

Stability is not complacency. A stable patient may need less intensive care while maintaining honest self-observation, support, medication, healthy routines, and readiness to respond.

Mature recovery is not constant fear. It is calm, accurate respect.

Deeper Therapeutic Work and Individualized Pacing

As recovery stabilizes, some patients may develop enough regulation, safety, readiness, and support to address unresolved grief, trauma-related symptoms, chronic anxiety or depression, painful relationship patterns, shame, chronic pain, sleep disorders, and other medical or psychiatric conditions. Other patients may appropriately begin elements of this work earlier. There is no universal sequence.

Earlier care may need to prioritize immediate safety, substance-use stabilization, sleep, and basic regulation, while still responding to trauma and grief in a trauma-informed manner. The depth and pacing of therapeutic work should be matched to the patient's current capacity for regulation, safety, readiness, preference, and support.

This work should occur with providers who understand both the underlying condition and the addictive illness and within a treatment context capable of responding if symptoms or recurrence risk increase.

Safety and stabilization can provide a foundation for deeper healing, but trauma and grief care should be individualized rather than rigidly deferred.

Recurrence as Information

If recurrence occurs, it should be taken seriously. It may reflect a combination of increased demand, reduced support, missed or rapidly emerging warning signs, inadequate treatment intensity for the conditions that developed, medication problems, environmental exposure, reduced honesty, or underestimated illness severity. Recurrence can also occur despite a thoughtful plan and does not prove one specific failure or mechanism.

Recurrence may indicate that the prior protection plan was insufficient for the conditions that developed and warrants serious reassessment.

The response should include immediate safety, compassionate accountability, reassessment, treatment adjustment, and repair of harm where needed rather than moral condemnation. Treatment intensity should rise when assessed risk and clinical need increase—not solely because a conceptual threshold is presumed to have been crossed.

Selected supporting evidence: [63–64,91].

Chapter 11 Closing Perspective

> *The goal is not perfect stability. It is earlier recognition, earlier disclosure, and earlier restoration of protection.*
>
> *A return to treatment is not a failure of recovery. It is one of the ways recovery protects itself.*

Chapter 12 asks what recovery is ultimately for: not only preventing recurrence, but restoring the freedom to live, connect, contribute, and accept responsibility.

Chapter Summary

Protecting remission depends on recognizing change before crisis, responding early, and maintaining a network of supports matched to the individual. Medication, monitoring, therapy, mutual support, sleep, stress management, cue management, relationships, and purpose may all contribute.

Key Clinical Takeaways

- Recurrence is often preceded by changes in sleep, stress, isolation, honesty, routine, cue exposure, or connection, although not every episode follows the same sequence.
- An early response plan should identify warning signs, disclosure pathways, and specific actions before judgment becomes less reliable.
- Twelve-Step Facilitation, Alcoholics Anonymous, and sponsorship are related but distinct; sponsors are nonprofessional peers, not clinicians or emergency services.
- The depth and pacing of trauma, grief, and other therapeutic work should be matched to current regulation, safety, readiness, preference, and support.

Chapter 12 — Living Beyond Survival

From Protected Recovery to Meaning, Growth, and Contribution

Recovery often begins with survival-oriented needs: safety, stabilization, distance from substances, and enough support to interrupt the illness. Within the Homeostatic Reserve Model, survival is an early priority rather than the final goal; individual recovery pathways vary.

As regulation becomes more durable, connection, competence, meaning, creativity, responsibility, and contribution may become more reliably available. This is a proposed direction of recovery, not a universal stage sequence.

> *Recovery does not end when the patient stops using. It expands when the patient becomes increasingly able to live.*

Selected supporting evidence: [57–59].

From Immediate Relief to a Meaningful Life

Addictive illness may narrow attention toward avoiding withdrawal, finding relief, managing consequences, concealing illness, and surviving distress. Recovery may gradually widen attention toward relationships, work, family, health, values, service, creativity, learning, spirituality, and the future.

> *Recovery widens life from the urgent search for relief toward the sustained pursuit of what matters.*

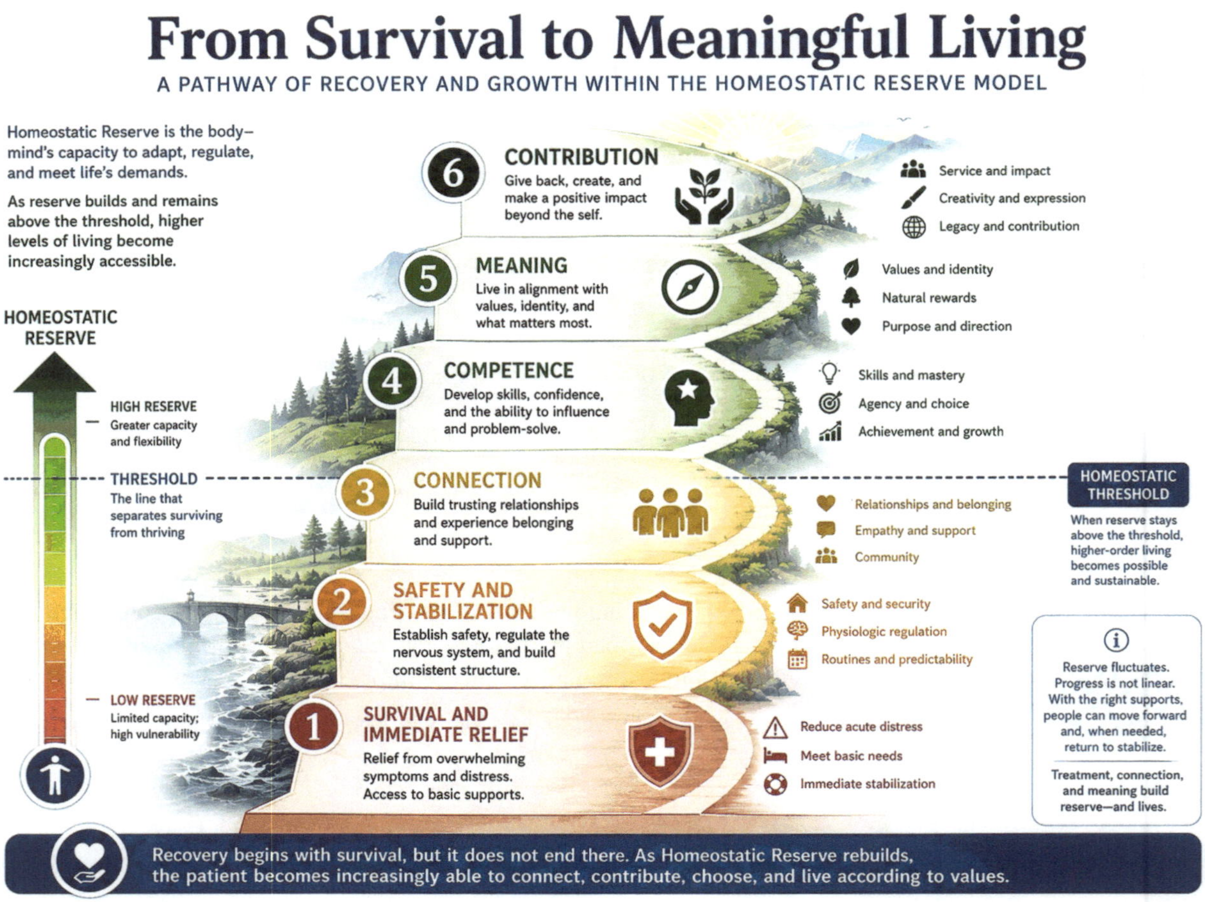

Figure 12.1. From Survival Toward Meaningful Living. Within the Homeostatic Reserve Model, rebuilding reserve may support movement from survival and stabilization toward connection, competence, meaning, creativity, contribution, and value-congruent living. The pathway is informed by Maslow's hierarchy while remaining non-rigid and individualized. This figure is a conceptual educational representation, not a validated stage model, outcome scale, or universal recovery sequence. Homeostatic Reserve represents integrated regulatory capacity, not a literal dopamine or neurotransmitter supply. Supporting evidence for component mechanisms: [57–58,82–83].

The Return of Choice

A central purpose of treatment is restoration of freedom. The patient may not become free from every craving, stressor, memory, consequence, or vulnerability. Within the model, treatment may restore enough capacity to pause, reflect, seek support, and act more consistently with long-term values.

> *Treatment does not choose for the patient. It can restore capacity so that the patient becomes increasingly able to choose and accept responsibility for those choices.*

Restored choice appears in ordinary moments: leaving a high-risk environment, telling the truth before confrontation, protecting sleep, asking for help, keeping a commitment, setting a boundary, or tolerating discomfort without escaping it.

Selected supporting evidence: [11,57,69].

The Person Is Not the Illness

People living with addictive illness retain dignity, personhood, and the capacity for recovery. Terminology matters in a field burdened by stigma. The manuscript uses person-first language: a person with alcohol use disorder, opioid use disorder, or another addictive illness—not an alcoholic or addict. Person-first language does not minimize risk, consequences, or the need for accountability.

> *A person has an illness. The person is not the illness.*

In the depths of illness, patients may describe themselves through the lens of consequences: a failed parent, damaged professional, untrustworthy spouse, or someone who disappointed the people they value most.

Some patients describe feeling that the illness changed them into someone they never intended to become. The statement may reflect profound pain about behavior sharply inconsistent with values and preferred identity. The consequences and harm are real and may require safety measures, accountability, changed behavior, restitution, and repair.

Treatment offers a more complete interpretation:

> *This is part of what happened while you were very sick. It requires honesty, accountability, safety, and repair, but it is not the whole truth of who you are.*

The anguish may itself reveal that values remain present. Pain can arise because behavior moved far from what the patient believes and wants life to represent. That understanding should support responsibility rather than shame-based identity collapse.

Within the Homeostatic Reserve Model, severe depletion and survival-oriented functioning may organize behavior around immediate relief more than identity, relationships, and long-term values. This can help explain diminished capacity without excusing harm or erasing agency.

Illness may help explain behavior, but it does not make harmful behavior acceptable. Recovery includes responsibility, safety, honest acknowledgment, changed action, and repair where possible.

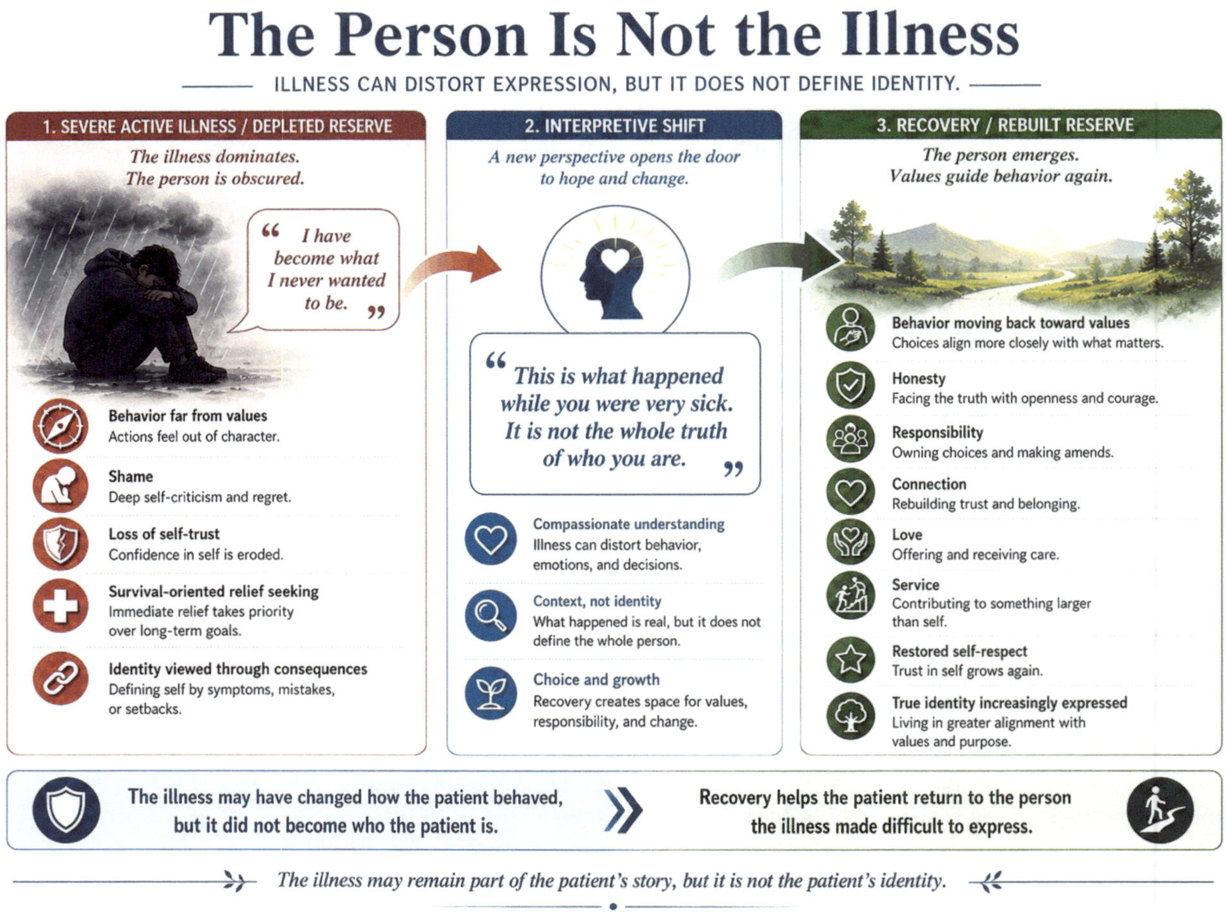

Figure 12.2. The Person Is Not the Illness. Severe illness may produce behavior far from the patient's values and lead to shame-based identity conclusions. Recovery may restore honesty, responsibility, safety, repair, connection, love, service, self-respect, and the capacity to express enduring values. This figure is a conceptual educational representation, not a diagnostic or moral classification. Homeostatic Reserve represents integrated regulatory capacity, not a literal dopamine or neurotransmitter supply. Supporting evidence for component mechanisms: [59,73–74].

Selected supporting evidence: [59,73–74].

Meaning Does Not Require Perfection

Patients sometimes believe meaningful living can begin only after every consequence is repaired. Some losses remain. Relationships may not fully recover. Professional roles may change. Legal or medical consequences may continue.

> *A meaningful life is not a life without loss. It is a life in which the patient can respond to loss without abandoning values or recovery.*

Selected supporting evidence: [58,89].

Connection, Competence, and Contribution

Recovery may be reflected in increasing capacity for connection. The patient may become more able to tolerate closeness, trust others, become emotionally available, repair relationships, accept support, and participate in community. These changes are important but not required in one uniform form or timetable.

Competence develops through work, parenting, education, service, managing health, keeping routines, and following through. Healthy competence is grounded in evidence rather than grandiosity.

Contribution may become a source of meaning. The patient may help family, peers, colleagues, patients, students, or others facing similar illness. Service is one possible pathway and should not be imposed as a requirement or substitute for treatment.

Within the model, service may strengthen recovery capacity through meaning, connection, gratitude, self-respect, identity, and perspective. “Filling the tank” remains a teaching metaphor, not a measured effect.

> *Service does not erase the past. It allows the past to become a source of understanding and contribution.*

Selected supporting evidence: [57,89–90].

Work, Success, and Sustainable Growth

Work may provide structure, identity, competence, income, contribution, and social connection. The goal is not simply to return to the prior role quickly. It is to return in a way compatible with health and recovery.

Success itself can become a stressor. Promotion, travel, recognition, increased responsibility, and financial improvement may reduce sleep, treatment, meetings, and family time.

> *Growth is sustainable only when its demands fit the patient’s current capacity.*

Selected supporting evidence: [57–58,60].

Natural Reward, Pleasure, and Meaning

As hedonic function and broader regulation improve, ordinary life may become more rewarding: food, music, exercise, nature, intimacy, humor, creativity, work, family, and quiet. Hedonic improvement is multidimensional and should not be inferred from dopamine level or D2/D3 receptor availability alone.

Natural reward may be less intense than intoxication but more integrated, sustainable, and consistent with the life the patient values.

Not every meaningful activity is immediately pleasurable. Parenting, treatment, work, exercise, grief work, making amends, and caring for health may be difficult.

> *Pleasure answers, “What feels good now?” Meaning asks, “What is worth doing even when it is difficult?”*

> *The ability to live an ordinary day without needing to escape it is a profound form of recovery.*

Selected supporting evidence: [6,14,58].

Grief, Repair, and Forgiveness

As patients heal, they may become more aware of lost time, health, relationships, opportunities, trust, career progression, or earlier versions of themselves.

Greater insight can initially bring greater pain. For some patients, that pain may be part of healing rather than evidence that recovery is failing; clinicians should also assess depression, trauma symptoms, suicide risk, and other conditions rather than assuming distress is therapeutic.

Repair may involve apology, restitution, changed behavior, consistency, accepting boundaries, and allowing others to decide what level of relationship is safe.

> *The patient is responsible for repair, but not entitled to a particular response.*

Forgiveness should not be forced and should never erase truth, consequence, or safety.

Spirituality, Creativity, and Transcendence

Some patients describe recovery as spiritual; others do not. Spirituality may involve faith, humility, awe, gratitude, service, connection, surrender of control, or commitment to values larger than immediate desire. Secular, cultural, philosophical, and relational sources of meaning are equally legitimate when they support health and responsibility.

Creativity may return as recovery deepens. Writing, music, building, cooking, gardening, studying, designing, or problem solving may support identity and natural reward, although recovery does not require any particular creative expression.

Selected supporting evidence: [57,89].

Freedom With Responsibility and Long-Term Care

As autonomy increases, responsibility remains central. Fewer restrictions and less intensive monitoring may require honest self-observation, continued support, medication adherence when indicated, attention to warning signs, and willingness to increase care when needed. The appropriate type, intensity, and duration of support vary by patient.

> *Freedom in recovery is not freedom from responsibility. It is the restored capacity to carry responsibility more reliably.*

A patient may live a rich and meaningful life while remaining vulnerable to recurrence. These are not contradictions.

> *Mature recovery does not require denying vulnerability. It incorporates vulnerability into wise living.*

Ongoing medication, therapy, monitoring, mutual-support meetings, sponsorship, physician care, or structured support should not automatically be interpreted as failure. Sustained treatment may be one reason stability is possible, while the specific combination and duration should remain diagnosis-, risk-, response-, and preference-sensitive.

Selected supporting evidence: [36,63–64].

From Fear of Loss Toward Love of Life

Early recovery may be organized partly around avoiding substances, consequences, loss of employment, or family pressure. For some patients, motivation later becomes increasingly organized around protecting health, relationships, freedom, identity, service, purpose, and meaning. External and internal motives can continue to coexist.

For some patients, the center of recovery may gradually shift from fear of loss toward love of life.

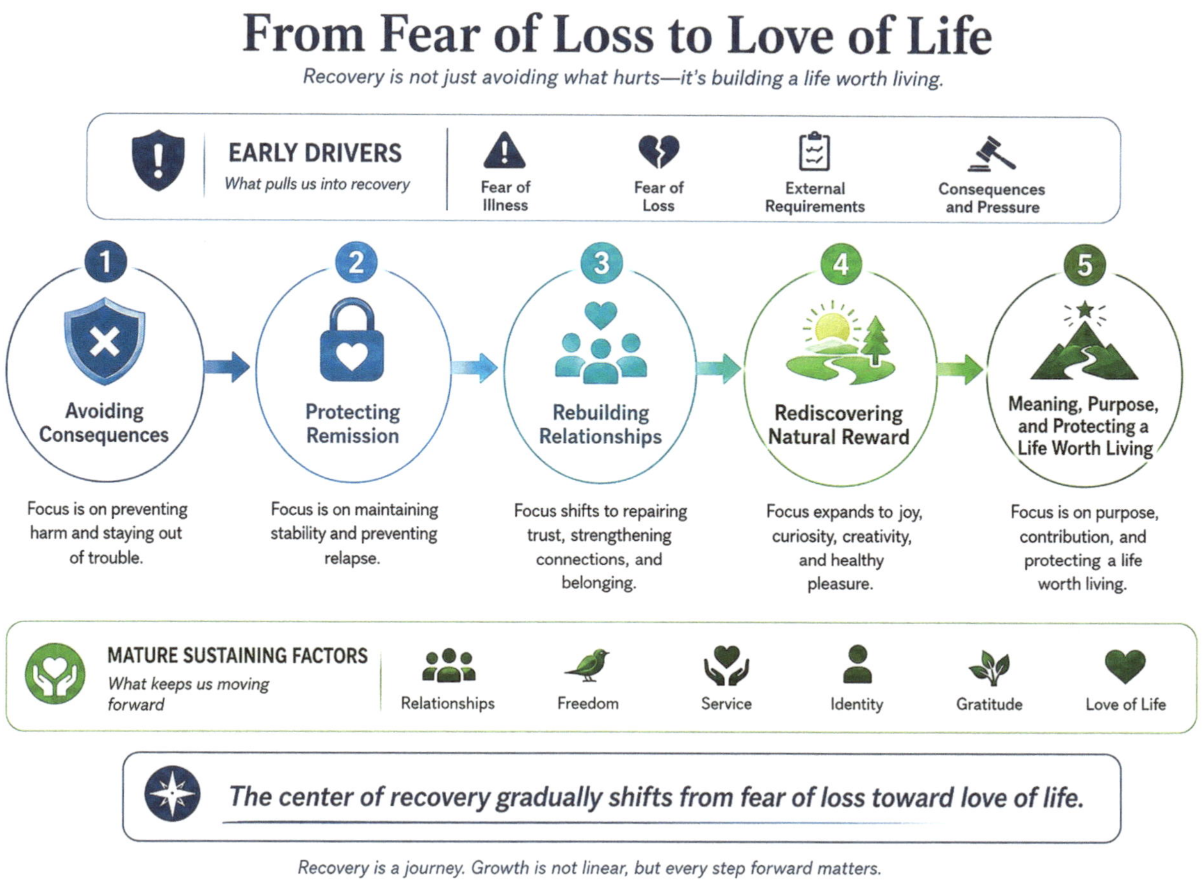

Figure 12.3. From Fear of Loss Toward Love of Life. Recovery motivation may evolve from avoiding consequences and protecting remission toward rediscovering natural reward, rebuilding relationships, living with purpose, and protecting a meaningful life. This is one possible conceptual pathway, not a required stage sequence or validated motivation scale. Homeostatic Reserve represents integrated regulatory capacity, not a literal dopamine or neurotransmitter supply. Supporting evidence for component mechanisms: [57–58,70].

Supporting evidence for component mechanisms: [57–58,70]. These sources support component mechanisms; the model's integrated relationship remains an original conceptual proposition.

Chapter 12 Closing Perspective

Recovery does not remove every challenge, but effective treatment helps restore the brain's capacity to engage in that fight.

Treatment makes the fight more fair.

Healing does not create goodness or values; it restores greater capacity to express them through responsible, accountable action.

The ultimate goal is not merely abstinence. It is restored freedom—the capacity to connect, contribute, choose, and live a meaningful life.

Chapter Summary

Recovery ultimately concerns the return of freedom: the capacity to connect, contribute, choose, repair, experience natural reward, tolerate difficulty, and organize life around meaning rather than immediate relief. The goal is not perfection but increasingly responsible, value-congruent living.

Key Clinical Takeaways

- The person is not the illness, but compassion does not remove accountability, boundaries, safety, or repair.
- Meaning, spirituality or secular purpose, creativity, work, service, and relationships may support recovery through different individual pathways.
- Long-term care should be individualized; ongoing support does not imply permanent incapacity or identical treatment intensity for every patient.
- Treatment does not choose values for the patient. It helps restore the capacity to live by them.

Glossary of Major Terms

Addictive illness

A chronic medical illness involving interacting genetic, developmental, environmental, psychiatric, learning, stress, motivational, and executive-control processes. The term emphasizes illness without reducing the person to the diagnosis.

Borrowed normality

A clinical description for the experience of a substance effect that may feel less like intoxication and more like access to calm, energy, focus, confidence, connection, or relief that the person cannot reliably access otherwise. It is not a validated diagnostic subtype or biomarker.

Congruence

Increasing alignment among thoughts, words, choices, behavior, and personally held values. Within the model, congruence is a recovery-relevant clinical process, not a laboratory measure.

Executive function

Cognitive capacities involved in attention, working memory, inhibition, planning, judgment, cognitive flexibility, and organizing behavior around future goals.

Hedonic tone

The broad capacity to experience pleasure, interest, positive engagement, and reward from ordinary life. Hedonic tone is influenced by multiple neural and psychological systems and is not a direct measure of dopamine.

Homeostasis

The capacity of a living system to maintain sufficient internal stability while adapting to changing demands. Homeostasis is dynamic regulation, not the absence of change.

Homeostatic Reserve Healing Trajectory

The temporal component of the model describing nonlinear, multidomain change in reserve, protection, function, and independence across treatment and recovery. Its phases and curves are heuristic rather than universal timetables.

Homeostatic Reserve

Within the Homeostatic Reserve Model, the person's dynamic, integrated functional capacity to maintain or regain regulation under stress. It reflects the resulting regulatory margin created by biological, psychiatric, cognitive, motivational, relational, environmental, coping, and meaning-based systems working together.

Homeostatic Threshold

The relatively stable conceptual boundary used within the model to describe a change in the relative availability of survival-oriented relief and value-congruent regulation. It is not a measured biological cutoff.

Integrated care

A coordinated approach in which addictive illness, co-occurring psychiatric and medical conditions, family and environmental factors, and recovery needs remain visible within one shared treatment formulation rather than being treated as unrelated problems.

Multidisciplinary treatment

Care in which professionals from several disciplines contribute distinct, coordinated functions. The necessary team varies by patient and may include medicine, nursing, psychotherapy, addiction counseling, group treatment, family therapy, peer support, case management, and other specialties.

Natural reward

Ordinary experiences—such as food, rest, relationships, mastery, play, creativity, service, spirituality or secular meaning, and contribution—that support motivation, learning, regulation, and engagement with life.

Negative reinforcement

Strengthening of a behavior because the behavior reduces or removes an aversive state. Negative reinforcement is not punishment.

Recovery capital

The internal and external resources available to support recovery, including personal, social, community, cultural, financial, housing, treatment, and relational resources.

Recovery Maintenance Network

The individualized set of treatments, people, routines, monitoring practices, environmental protections, and sources of meaning that help protect remission over time.

Reserve–Threshold–Trajectory architecture

The model's central organization: Reserve describes changing integrated capacity; Threshold describes conceptual functional position; Trajectory describes change across time.

Stage-matched care

The model-informed principle that treatment methods, intensity, directness, and depth should be matched to the patient's current safety, regulation, functional capacity, preferences, supports, and movement along the Healing Trajectory rather than to time alone.

Structure as borrowed reserve

The model's teaching metaphor for the way predictable routines, monitoring, access reduction, sleep opportunity, meals, accountability, and organized care can temporarily supply external support when internal regulation is unreliable.

Survival-oriented vulnerability

A below-threshold functional state in which urgency, withdrawal, stress, conditioned motivation, and immediate relief gain disproportionate influence over behavior.

Team coherence

A shared clinical formulation and coordinated plan in which different disciplines reinforce one understandable path through care rather than sending contradictory or disconnected messages.

Therapeutic pacing

Matching the depth, intensity, and timing of questioning, feedback, trauma work, grief work, and other interventions to the patient's current capacity for safety, regulation, emotional tolerance, and integration.

Treatment scaffolding

External and biological supports that help stabilize behavior and regulation while recovery capacity is rebuilding. Structure may scaffold behavior from the outside; medication may scaffold regulation from the inside.

Unfair Fight

Within the model, the disproportionate advantage held by immediate, conditioned, survival-oriented relief over healthy alternatives when reserve is low. The proposition does not imply absent agency or remove accountability.

Value-congruent regulation

A functional state in which reflection, support, emotional regulation, natural reward, long-term consequences, and personally held values are sufficiently available to guide behavior more reliably.

Withdrawal management

The medical and clinical management of intoxication and withdrawal risk. It is a phase of treatment and should not be mistaken for complete treatment of the underlying addictive illness.

References

1. Cannon WB. Organization for physiological homeostasis. Physiol Rev. 1929;9(3):399-431. doi:10.1152/physrev.1929.9.3.399.
2. McEwen BS, Stellar E. Stress and the individual: mechanisms leading to disease. Arch Intern Med. 1993;153(18):2093-2101. PMID 8379800.
3. Stern Y. Cognitive reserve. Neuropsychologia. 2009;47(10):2015-2028. PMID 19467352; doi:10.1016/j.neuropsychologia.2009.03.004.
4. Bandinelli S, et al. Frailty and the homeostatic network. Mech Ageing Dev. 2010;131(7-8):502-504. PMID 20518187.
5. Fried LP, et al. The physical frailty syndrome as a transition from homeostatic symphony to cacophony. Nat Aging. 2021;1:36-46. PMID 34476409.
6. Berridge KC, Robinson TE. Liking, wanting, and the incentive-sensitization theory of addiction. Am Psychol. 2016;71(8):670-679. PMID 27977239; doi:10.1037/amp0000059.
7. Schultz W, Dayan P, Montague PR. A neural substrate of prediction and reward. Science. 1997;275(5306):1593-1599. PMID 9054347.
8. Salamone JD, Correa M. The mysterious motivational functions of mesolimbic dopamine. Neuron. 2012;76(3):470-485. PMID 23141060.
9. Volkow ND, Michaelides M, Baler R. The neuroscience of drug reward and addiction. Physiol Rev. 2019;99(4):2115-2140. PMID 31507244; doi:10.1152/physrev.00014.2018.
10. Koob GF, Volkow ND. Neurobiology of addiction: a neurocircuitry analysis. Lancet Psychiatry. 2016;3(8):760-773. PMID 27475769.
11. Goldstein RZ, Volkow ND. Dysfunction of the prefrontal cortex in addiction: neuroimaging findings and clinical implications. Nat Rev Neurosci. 2011;12(11):652-669. PMID 22011681.
12. Robinson TE, Berridge KC. The neural basis of drug craving: an incentive-sensitization theory of addiction. Brain Res Brain Res Rev. 1993;18(3):247-291. PMID 8401595.
13. Treadway MT, Zald DH. Reconsidering anhedonia in depression: lessons from translational neuroscience. Neurosci Biobehav Rev. 2011;35(3):537-555. PMID 20603146.
14. Berridge KC, Kringelbach ML. Pleasure systems in the brain. Neuron. 2015;86(3):646-664. PMID 25950633.
15. Volkow ND, Fowler JS, Wang GJ, Baler R, Telang F. Imaging dopamine's role in drug abuse and addiction. Neuropharmacology. 2009;56 Suppl 1:3-8. PMID 18617195.
16. Pavlov IP. Conditioned Reflexes: An Investigation of the Physiological Activity of the Cerebral Cortex. Oxford: Oxford University Press; 1927. Book.
17. O'Doherty J, Dayan P, Schultz J, Deichmann R, Friston K, Dolan RJ. Dissociable roles of ventral and dorsal striatum in instrumental conditioning. Science. 2004;304(5669):452-454. PMID 15087550.
18. Everitt BJ, Robbins TW. Drug addiction: updating actions to habits to compulsions ten years on. Annu Rev Psychol. 2016;67:23-50. PMID 26253543.
19. Maier SU, Makwana AB, Hare TA. Acute stress impairs self-control in goal-directed choice by altering multiple functional connections within the brain's decision circuits. Neuron. 2015;87(3):621-631. PMID 26247866.
20. Yoo SS, Gujar N, Hu P, Jolesz FA, Walker MP. The human emotional brain without sleep—a prefrontal amygdala disconnect. Curr Biol. 2007;17(20):R877-R878. PMID 17956744.
21. Verhulst B, Neale MC, Kendler KS. The heritability of alcohol use disorders: a meta-analysis of twin and adoption studies. Psychol Med. 2015;45(5):1061-1072. PMID 25171596.
22. Goldman D, Oroszi G, Ducci F. The genetics of addictions: uncovering the genes. Nat Rev Genet. 2005;6(7):521-532. PMID 15995696.
23. Dube SR, Felitti VJ, Dong M, Chapman DP, Giles WH, Anda RF. Childhood abuse, neglect, and household dysfunction and the risk of illicit drug use. Pediatrics. 2003;111(3):564-572. PMID 12612237.
24. Hughes K, Bellis MA, Hardcastle KA, et al. The effect of multiple adverse childhood experiences on health: a systematic review and meta-analysis. Lancet Public Health. 2017;2(8):e356-e366. PMID 29253477.
25. Sinha R. Chronic stress, drug use, and vulnerability to addiction. Ann N Y Acad Sci. 2008;1141:105-130. PMID 18991954.
26. Lai HMX, Cleary M, Sitharthan T, Hunt GE. Prevalence of comorbid substance use, anxiety and mood disorders in epidemiological surveys, 1990-2014: a systematic review and meta-analysis. Drug Alcohol Depend. 2015;154:1-13. PMID 26072219; doi:10.1016/j.drugalcdep.2015.05.031.
27. Samaha AN, Robinson TE. Why does the rapid delivery of drugs to the brain promote addiction? Trends Pharmacol Sci. 2005;26(2):82-87. PMID 15681025.

28. Koob GF, Le Moal M. Drug addiction, dysregulation of reward, and allostasis. Neuropsychopharmacology. 2001;24(2):97-129. PMID 11120394.

29. Koob GF, Le Moal M. Drug abuse: hedonic homeostatic dysregulation. Science. 1997;278(5335):52-58. PMID 9311926.

30. Gardner EL. Addiction and brain reward and antireward pathways. Adv Psychosom Med. 2011;30:22-60. PMID 21508625.

31. Goldstein RZ, Craig AD, Bechara A, et al. The neurocircuitry of impaired insight in drug addiction. Trends Cogn Sci. 2009;13(9):372-380. PMID 19716751.

32. American Society of Addiction Medicine. The ASAM Criteria, Fourth Edition: official overview, assessment guides, and implementation resources. Rockville, MD: ASAM; 2023-2026. Official standard; accessed 2026-07-14.

33. American Psychiatric Association. Diagnostic and Statistical Manual of Mental Disorders. 5th ed, text rev. Washington, DC: American Psychiatric Association Publishing; 2022. ISBN 978-0-89042-575-6.

34. American Society of Addiction Medicine. The ASAM Clinical Practice Guideline on Alcohol Withdrawal Management. J Addict Med. 2020;14(3S Suppl 1):1-72. Official clinical guideline.

35. American Society of Addiction Medicine and partner societies. Joint Clinical Practice Guideline on Benzodiazepine Tapering. Rockville, MD: ASAM; 2025. Official clinical guideline; accessed 2026-07-14.

36. Substance Abuse and Mental Health Services Administration. TIP 63: Medications for Opioid Use Disorder. Updated 2021. Rockville, MD: SAMHSA; 2021. PEP21-02-01-002.

37. American Society of Addiction Medicine. National Practice Guideline for the Treatment of Opioid Use Disorder: 2020 Focused Update. J Addict Med. 2020;14(2S Suppl 1):1-91. Official clinical guideline.

38. American Society of Addiction Medicine, American Academy of Addiction Psychiatry. Clinical Practice Guideline on the Management of Stimulant Use Disorder. J Addict Med. 2024;18(1S Suppl 1):1-56. Official clinical guideline.

39. McPheeters M, et al. Pharmacotherapy for Alcohol Use Disorder: a systematic review and meta-analysis. JAMA. 2023;330(17):1653-1665. PMID 37934220.

40. Mattick RP, Breen C, Kimber J, Davoli M. Buprenorphine maintenance versus placebo or methadone maintenance for opioid dependence. Cochrane Database Syst Rev. 2014;(2):CD002207. PMID 24500948.

41. Sordo L, Barrio G, Bravo MJ, et al. Mortality risk during and after opioid substitution treatment: systematic review and meta-analysis of cohort studies. BMJ. 2017;357:j1550. PMID 28446428.

42. Lee JD, Nunes EV Jr, Novo P, et al. Comparative effectiveness of extended-release naltrexone versus buprenorphine-naloxone for opioid relapse prevention (X:BOT). Lancet. 2018;391(10118):309-318. PMID 29150198.

43. Kakko J, Svanborg KD, Kreek MJ, Heilig M. One-year retention and social function after buprenorphine-assisted relapse prevention treatment for heroin dependence. Lancet. 2003;361(9358):662-668. PMID 12606177.

44. Lee JD, Friedmann PD, Kinlock TW, et al. Extended-release naltrexone to prevent opioid relapse in criminal justice offenders. N Engl J Med. 2016;374(13):1232-1242. PMID 27028913.

45. Leone FT, Zhang Y, Evers-Casey S, et al. Initiating pharmacologic treatment in tobacco-dependent adults: an official American Thoracic Society clinical practice guideline. Am J Respir Crit Care Med. 2020;202(2):e5-e31. PMID 32663106.

46. Ronsley C, Nolan S, Knight R, et al. Treatment of stimulant use disorder: a systematic review of reviews. PLoS One. 2020;15(6):e0234809. PMID 32555667; doi:10.1371/journal.pone.0234809.

47. Stavro K, Pelletier J, Potvin S. Widespread and sustained cognitive deficits in alcoholism: a meta-analysis. Addict Biol. 2013;18(2):203-213. PMID 22264351.

48. Scott JC, Woods SP, Matt GE, et al. Neurocognitive effects of methamphetamine: a critical review and meta-analysis. Neuropsychol Rev. 2007;17(3):275-297. PMID 17694436.

49. Crean RD, Crane NA, Mason BJ. An evidence based review of acute and long-term effects of cannabis use on executive cognitive functions. J Addict Med. 2011;5(1):1-8. PMID 21321675.

50. Heilbronner RL, Sweet JJ, Morgan JE, Larrabee GJ, Millis SR. American Academy of Clinical Neuropsychology consensus conference statement on the neuropsychological assessment of effort, response bias, and malingering. Clin Neuropsychol. 2009;23(7):1093-1129. PMID 19735055; doi:10.1080/13854040903155063.

51. Koob GF. A role for brain stress systems in addiction. Neuron. 2008;59(1):11-34. PMID 18614026.

52. Durazzo TC, Mon A, Gazdzinski S, et al. Serial longitudinal MRI data indicate non-linear regional gray matter volume recovery in abstinent alcohol-dependent individuals. Addict Biol. 2015;20(5):956-967. PMID 25170881.

53. Bates ME, Buckman JF, Nguyen TT. The mean and the individual: integrating variable-centered and person-specific analyses of cognitive recovery in alcohol use disorder. Front Psychiatry. 2013;4:177. PMID 24399976.

54. Charlet K, Rosenthal A, Lohoff FW, Heinz A, Beck A. Imaging resilience and recovery in alcohol dependence. Addiction. 2018;113(10):1933-1950. PMID 29744956.

55. Brower KJ. Insomnia, alcoholism and relapse. Sleep Med Rev. 2003;7(6):523-539. PMID 15018094.

56. Linke SE, Ussher M. Exercise-based treatments for substance use disorders: evidence, theory, and practicality. Am J Drug Alcohol Abuse. 2015;41(1):7-15. PMID 25397661.

57. Inanlou M, Bahmani B, Farhoudian A, Rafiee F. Addiction recovery: a systematic review. Iran J Psychiatry. 2020;15(2):172-181. PMID 32426014.

58. Laudet AB. The case for considering quality of life in addiction research and clinical practice. Addict Sci Clin Pract. 2011;6(1):44-55. PMID 22003421.

59. Betty Ford Institute Consensus Panel. What is recovery? A working definition from the Betty Ford Institute. J Subst Abuse Treat. 2007;33(3):221-228. PMID 17889294.

60. Cloud W, Granfield R. Conceptualizing recovery capital: expansion of a theoretical construct. Subst Use Misuse. 2008;43(12-13):1971-1986. PMID 19016174.

61. Vilsaint CL, Kelly JF, Bergman BG, et al. Development and validation of a Brief Assessment of Recovery Capital (BARC-10) for alcohol and drug use disorder. Addiction. 2017;112(12):2231-2242. PMID 28578224.

62. Best D, et al. The science of recovery capital: where do we go from here? Addiction. 2022;117(4):1139-1145. PMID 34729852.

63. McKay JR. Impact of continuing care on recovery from substance use disorder. Alcohol Res. 2021;41(1):01. PMID 33500871.

64. McLellan AT, Lewis DC, O'Brien CP, Kleber HD. Drug dependence, a chronic medical illness: implications for treatment, insurance, and outcomes evaluation. JAMA. 2000;284(13):1689-1695. PMID 11015800.

65. Substance Abuse and Mental Health Services Administration. TIP 41: Substance Abuse Treatment: Group Therapy. Rockville, MD: SAMHSA; 2005, updated online 2015. HHS Publication SMA15-3991.

66. Eddie D, Hoffman L, Vilsaint C, et al. Lived experience in new models of care for substance use disorder: a systematic review of peer recovery support services and recovery coaching. Front Psychol. 2019;10:1052. PMID 31263434.

67. Kelly JF, Humphreys K, Ferri M. Alcoholics Anonymous and other 12-step programs for alcohol use disorder. Cochrane Database Syst Rev. 2020;3(3):CD012880. PMID 32159228.

68. National Institute on Alcohol Abuse and Alcoholism. Mutual-Support Groups and Recovery Support. Bethesda, MD: NIAAA; current web guidance. Official guidance; accessed 2026-07-14.

69. Substance Abuse and Mental Health Services Administration. TIP 35: Enhancing Motivation for Change in Substance Use Disorder Treatment. Rockville, MD: SAMHSA; 2019. PEP19-02-01-003.

70. Urbanoski KA, Wild TC. Assessing self-determined motivation for addiction treatment: validity of the Treatment Entry Questionnaire. J Subst Abuse Treat. 2012;43(1):70-79. PMID 22138201.

71. Substance Abuse and Mental Health Services Administration. TIP 57: Trauma-Informed Care in Behavioral Health Services. Rockville, MD: SAMHSA; 2014. HHS Publication SMA14-4816.

72. Roberts NP, Roberts PA, Jones N, Bisson JI. Psychological interventions for post-traumatic stress disorder and comorbid substance use disorder: a systematic review and meta-analysis. Clin Psychol Rev. 2015;38:25-38. PMID 25792193; doi:10.1016/j.cpr.2015.02.007.

73. Kelly JF, Westerhoff CM. Does it matter how we refer to individuals with substance-related conditions? A randomized study of two commonly used terms. Int J Drug Policy. 2010;21(3):202-207. PMID 20005692.

74. National Institute on Drug Abuse. Words Matter: Preferred Language for Talking About Addiction. Bethesda, MD: NIDA; current web guidance. Official guidance; accessed 2026-07-14.

75. McLellan AT, Skipper GS, Campbell M, DuPont RL. Five year outcomes in a cohort study of physicians treated for substance use disorders in the United States. BMJ. 2008;337:a2038. PMID 18984632.

76. DuPont RL, McLellan AT, Carr G, Gendel M, Skipper GE. How are addicted physicians treated? A national survey of physician health programs. J Subst Abuse Treat. 2009;37(1):1-7. PMID 19161896.

77. Federal Aviation Administration. Guide for Aviation Medical Examiners, including HIMS drug and alcohol certification materials. Washington, DC: FAA; current edition updated 2026. Official aeromedical standard; accessed 2026-07-14.

78. U.S. Department of Transportation. 49 CFR Part 40—Procedures for Transportation Workplace Drug and Alcohol Testing Programs, including SAP, return-to-duty, and follow-up testing provisions. Washington, DC: DOT; current through 2026. Official federal regulation; accessed 2026-07-14.

79. Federation of State Physician Health Programs. Physician Health Program Guidelines and Public Policy Resources. Washington, DC: FSPHP; current web resources. Professional guidance; accessed 2026-07-14.

80. Florida Legislature. Florida Statutes §456.076: Impaired practitioner programs. Tallahassee, FL: State of Florida; current 2026 statute. Official state law; accessed 2026-07-14.

81. U.S. Department of Health and Human Services. Confidentiality of Substance Use Disorder Patient Records, 42 CFR Part 2; 2024 Final Rule and current compliance resources. Washington, DC: HHS. Official federal regulation; accessed 2026-07-14.

82. Maslow AH. A theory of human motivation. Psychol Rev. 1943;50(4):370-396. doi:10.1037/h0054346.

83. Maslow AH. Motivation and Personality. New York, NY: Harper & Brothers; 1954. Book.

84. Volkow ND, Wang GJ, Telang F, et al. Cocaine cues and dopamine in dorsal striatum: mechanism of craving in cocaine addiction. J Neurosci. 2006;26(24):6583-6588. PMID 16775146.

85. Childress AR, Ehrman RN, Wang Z, et al. Prelude to passion: limbic activation by "unseen" drug and sexual cues. PLoS One. 2008;3(1):e1506. PMID 18231593.

86. Bergman BG, Kelly JF. Online digital recovery support services: an overview of the science and their potential to help individuals with substance use disorder during COVID-19 and beyond. J Subst Abuse Treat. 2021;120:108152. PMID 33129636.

87. Reif S, George P, Braude L, et al. Recovery housing: assessing the evidence. Psychiatr Serv. 2014;65(3):295-300. PMID 24226305.

88. Substance Abuse and Mental Health Services Administration. TIP 39: Substance Use Disorder Treatment and Family Therapy. Rockville, MD: SAMHSA; updated 2020. PEP20-02-02-004.

89. Laudet AB, Morgen K, White WL. The role of social supports, spirituality, religiousness, life meaning and affiliation with 12-step fellowships in quality of life satisfaction among individuals in recovery. Alcohol Treat Q. 2006;24(1-2):33-73. PMID 16892161.

90. Mawson E, Best D, Beckwith M, Dingle GA, Lubman DI. Social identity, social networks and recovery capital in emerging adulthood: a pilot study. Subst Abuse Treat Prev Policy. 2015;10:45. PMID 26560076.

91. Witkiewitz K, Marlatt GA. Relapse prevention for alcohol and drug problems: that was Zen, this is Tao. Am Psychol. 2004;59(4):224-235. PMID 15149263.

92. Substance Abuse and Mental Health Services Administration. TIP 42: Substance Use Disorder Treatment for People With Co-Occurring Disorders. Rockville, MD: SAMHSA; updated 2020. PEP20-02-01-004.

93. Alcoholics Anonymous World Services. Questions and Answers on Sponsorship. New York, NY: AA World Services; current pamphlet. Official fellowship pamphlet; accessed 2026-07-14.

94. National Institute on Drug Abuse. Principles of Drug Addiction Treatment: A Research-Based Guide. 3rd ed. Bethesda, MD: NIDA; 2018. NIH Publication 18-4180.

95. Saper CB, Chou TC, Elmquist JK. The need to feed: homeostatic and hedonic control of eating. Neuron. 2002;36(2):199-211. doi:10.1016/S0896-6273(02)00969-8. PMID 12383777.

96. Zimmerman CA, Leib DE, Knight ZA. Neural circuits underlying thirst and fluid homeostasis. Nat Rev Neurosci. 2017;18(8):459-469. doi:10.1038/nrn.2017.71. PMID 28638120.

97. Substance Abuse and Mental Health Services Administration. The Importance of Family Therapy in Substance Use Disorder Treatment. Advisory. Rockville, MD: SAMHSA; 2021. Publication No. PEP20-02-02-016.

98. Meier PS, Barrowclough C, Donmall MC. The role of the therapeutic alliance in the treatment of substance misuse: a critical review of the literature. Addiction. 2005;100(3):304-316. PMID 15733244; doi:10.1111/j.1360-0443.2004.00935.x.

99. Substance Abuse and Mental Health Services Administration. TIP 59: Improving Cultural Competence. Rockville, MD: SAMHSA; 2014. HHS Publication No. SMA14-4849.

100. Gropper J. A Guide to Growing Up—Addiction Recovery. 2nd ed. [Publisher not identified]; 2017. Short direct quotation used with permission of the author; publication page not supplied.

About the Author

Jeremy Mirabile, MD, ABPM-ADM, FASAM, is a physician whose clinical work has focused on the evaluation and treatment of substance use disorders, co-occurring psychiatric conditions, multidimensional treatment planning, and recovery in patients with complex clinical and professional responsibilities. Drawing on more than two decades of clinical experience, he developed the Homeostatic Reserve Model as an educational framework for explaining changing functional capacity during addictive illness, treatment, and recovery.

His teaching emphasizes that addiction is a medical illness rather than a moral identity; that severity should guide the structure and intensity of care; and that recovery extends beyond abstinence toward restored regulation, responsibility, relationships, purpose, and meaningful living.

Index

www.ingramcontent.com/pod-product-compliance
Lightning Source LLC
LaVergne TN
LVHW070936210926
848482LV00003B/254
* 9 7 9 8 9 9 7 2 0 0 3 0 5 *